Exclusively Female

"Women must assume responsibility for their bodies. No one else can—not the government, not the food industries, not even the family physician. In gaining control over one's health plan, the first priority is education. This, then, is the intention of the writer— to educate women on the mechanics of the menstrual cycle, to inform them as to possible nutritional reasons for an unbalanced and painful cycle, and to provide them with a natural, safe, and effective method of treating the problem."

From the Book

"Prior to reading *Exclusively Female* I had suffered from most of the PMS symptoms with increasing intensity since the beginning of my menstrual years. Since I started using the nutritional approach advocated by Ms. Ojeda, I have been able to give up the pain pills. The monthly suffering and the complete dissociation from my true self is gone, and I have begun to experience the happiness of being myself *every* day of the month."

S.C., *Fullerton, CA*

About the Author

Linda Ojeda is a writer and lecturer, specializing in topics which deal with the proper understanding and nutritional treatment of women's health problems.

Because her books and articles discuss these health issues in non-technical terms they are used extensively by professionals in the medical and health counseling fields, as well as by women who may be suffering the effects of these problems.

Ms. Ojeda is a frequent speaker at women's centers and conferences. She is a founding member of the Tree Of Life Seminars group, which sponsors and presents seminars on all aspects of the evolution of the female role in today's society.

Born in Jamestown, New York, Ms. Ojeda received her undergraduate training in Food & Nutrition at California State Polytechnic University, Pomona, and a Master of Science degree from Donsbach University, School of Nutrition. She is a member of several professional associations, including the American Medical Writers Association, the International Academy of Nutrition Consultants, and the National Health Federation. She now lives in Fullerton, California, managing a career, a husband, and two teenage children, and is currently researching and writing a book on menopause.

EXCLUSIVELY FEMALE

by Linda Ojeda

A Nutrition Guide for Better Menstrual Health

Hunter House

2nd (revised) edition published in 1983 by
Hunter House Inc., Publishers
PO Box 1302
Claremont, Ca 91711
ISBN 0-89793-032-0
Library of Congress Card Number: LC 83-081702

Cover design by Qalagraphia
Set in 11 on 12 point Goudy Old Style
Printed and bound in the USA

Dedicated to my daughter Jill

May her generation be more actively
involved in their own health care.

Notes on Using This Book

Exclusively Female contains a description of the menstrual cycle and common menstrual irregularities, together with suggestions for the nutritional treatment of these symptoms. In your study and use of this book for reference and self-help, the following information about where to find things may be useful:

Physiological—Various charts and figures are used in Chapter One (pp. 5–7) to describe the physiological mechanism and the complicated hormonal feedback system that controls menstruation. At the end of the book, on p. 97, there is a diagram of the female body showing the location of the glands that directly and indirectly affect the process.

Vitamin/Mineral Program—Specific vitamin and mineral supplements are suggested throughout the book, and a complete supplement program is outlined in Appendix A (pp. 105–121).

Food Source Listings—Food sources for the vitamins and minerals recommended are listed in Appendix B (pp. 122–27), so that women can incorporate more nutrient-rich foods into their diets.

Glossary—A glossary of the medical, physiological, or scientific terms used in the text has been included, starting on p. 97. The words listed are italicized where they first appear in the text.

Book References—Reference numbers, shown in parentheses in the text, refer to sources being quoted or used. These are numbered in sequence starting at the beginning of each chapter. A complete bibliography listing all these references is given on pp. 89–95.

IMPORTANT NOTE

The information contained in this book
is primarily for educational purposes.
The author neither diagnoses problems
nor prescribes specific remedies.
Women who suffer from menstrual
problems should use this information in
cooperation with their doctors
(hopefully nutrition-oriented ones). In
the event women choose to experiment
on their own, which is their right, they
must assume total responsibility.

Contents

List of Figures and Charts

Opening Statement

THE "CURSE" CAN BE BROKEN

BY ADOPTING

CERTAIN BASIC PRINCIPLES

✱ Menstrual discomfort is women's most common physical problem, but it is neither normal, natural, or necessary.

✱ Menstrual problems reveal a hormonal imbalance that can be the result of nutritional deficiencies.

✱ Proper nutrition can relieve the symptoms of menstruation by treating the actual cause of the problem.

✱ Nutrients seek to establish balance to the body.

✱ Not only are nutrients safe but they are also effective.

Acknowledgments

I am grateful to Linda Meoli who patiently listened to my ideas as we jogged and subsequently became my number one promoter.

Thank you to Donsbach University, School of Nutrition, for providing me with the incentive to research women's problems.

Special thanks to my dear friend Nancy McCulloch Graff for taking time from her summer vacation to edit the first edition of the book, and to Prem Sharma, who helped with the typesetting and publishing.

And finally to my husband, Roland, I am grateful for his recommendations and encouragement.

Introduction

Menstruation is a completely natural process and women experience it for many years of their lives. Yet for a great number of ladies it is a virtual nightmare. **Menstrual distress is so predominant, in fact, that it is known throughout the world as women's most common physical problem, with symptoms ranging from mild discomfort to severe mental anguish.** Traditionally, the attitude has been to either ignore the complaint or dismiss it as a "figment of the imagination." Many people, men in particular, have written it off as the "fate of womanhood," rejecting the need for treatment. And women have resigned themselves to endure their suffering in silence rather than face the skeptical responses that are so common.

Incredible as it may sound, even today women are being led to believe their problems are normal, and therefore must be accepted and endured. But **monthly pain is not normal, natural, or necessary.** It is a sign that something within the body is not functioning correctly and needs immediate attention: it is Nature's cry for help. The feelings of discomfort that women often experience may be an indication that their general health is inadequate, or that something specific is wrong.

Until recently, the male-dominated medical community adhered to the psychological theory of menstrual distress. Physicians freely handed out tranquilizers as the solace for all monthly ills. Even today, when a physical cause has been recognized, doctors still repeatedly choose to treat this natural event with a barrage of multicolored pills. Diuretics, painkillers, tranquilizers, and hormones are all prescribed to minimize monthly symptoms. The main drawback of this philosophy is that relief is temporary, and every month the drugs must be repeated. Over the course of several years, side effects from these chemicals may prove to be even more of a health hazard than the original problem.

While it still may not be universally accepted by male physicians, it has now been proven that **menstrual problems are real, and are not just a psychological escape. They are the result of a definite physical or biochemical malfunction.** For any number of reasons the body is secreting too much of one or more hormones and not enough of others, creating a hormonal imbalance. It is this imbalance that leads to an increase in a chemical substance called *prostaglandin,* which produces the physical pain as well as the mental symptoms related to menstruation. This same disturbance also forces other systems and organs to overcompensate, leading again to many disorders characteristically associated with the menstrual period.

The initial imbalance may be caused by several factors or combinations of factors. It could stem from a genetic predisposition, an organic malfunction, a vitamin or mineral deficiency, drugs, chemicals, stress, or any combination of these. Because of the possibility of there being a functional problem, it is always wise to consult a gynecologist first.

More often than not, however, menstrual difficulties are not organically induced, but are the result of nutritional deficiencies. Because an irregular cycle often reflects the general state of a woman's health, continuous monthly discomfort strongly suggests that a change in diet is needed.

Women in the United States are not as well nourished as they think. Even those women who conscientiously select a well-balanced diet can still be the victims of malnutrition. The internationally known nutritionist Dr. Carlton Fredericks states that "If we are to appraise the nutrition of American women by the changes in the menstrual disturbances when nutrition is bettered, we must come to the conclusion that most of them are poorly fed."

Proper nutrition or the right combination of nutrients can not only relieve the symptoms of menstruation, it can also treat the actual cause of the problem. By feeding the body the nutrients it needs, in the correct amount and concentration, one can re-establish hormone balance, maintain prostaglandins at the necessary ratios, and alleviate if not totally eliminate pain. Correct nutrition relieves the symptoms of menstruation by treating the actual source of the problem.

The objective of nutritional therapy is always to treat the whole person. The human body is extremely complex and one cannot deal with just one part of it without affecting other parts as well. The entire system operates harmoniously as a unit; therefore, to regulate the hormones within the cycle requires adjustment of the total body chemistry.

This is not a simple task. Every body is unique. The combination of nutrients that balances one person's chemistry may be ineffective in regulating another's. For this reason, it is imperative that women examine their own bodies, their individual genetic traits, life-styles, habits, and symptoms, so they can find the specific formula they need for pain-free menstruation.

Women must assume responsibility for their bodies. No one else can—not the government, not the food industries, not even the family physician. In gaining control over one's health plan, the first priority is education. This then is the intention of the writer—to educate women on the mechanics of the menstrual cycle, to inform them as to possible nutritional reasons for an unbalanced and painful cycle, and to provide them with a natural, safe, and effective method of treating the problem.

The studies included in this book have been taken primarily from researchers and scientists in the field of medicine and nutrition. While they provide the information that is needed, results come only when such information is applied.

1

Defining Menstruation

Compared to the process, the purpose of menstruation is uncomplicated. The monthly cycle quite simply allows for reproduction to occur. Each month a woman's body prepares to conceive, carry, and nourish a baby. In preparation for the event many simultaneous changes occur: an egg is produced, various hormones are secreted, and the lining of the uterus becomes thick. If the woman does not become pregnant the useless uterine lining is sloughed off through the vagina. The period of time in which this blood-like discharge occurs is called menstruation.

Menstruation has been described in many different ways. The Boston Women's Health Collective in their book *Our Bodies, Ourselves* picturesquely describe the process as "a tree shedding its leaves in the fall." Hilary Maddux, in her book on menstruation, portrays it as the "weeping of a disappointed uterus," in that discharge is the result of conception not having taken place in the previous cycle. The majority of women, however, do not view the cycle so poetically. Many find it an inconvenience, and for several it can be a trauma.

For the sake of simplicity, a 28-day cycle is used in de-

1

scribing the menstrual process. Although this is considered the classical textbook menstrual period, it is not the time schedule that most women follow. In fact, probably fewer than ten percent of women in their peak reproductive years actually have regular 28-day cycles. (1)   A cycle may extend from 21 to 40 days and still be considered physiologically normal. Even if it is 20 days one month and 43 days the next, it may be normal for some women. Variation is more often the rule than the exception.

Chain of Events

The menstrual system involves four different and independent structures (hypothalamus, pituitary, ovaries, and uterus) as well as three physiological processes (development of the egg resulting in ovulation, changes in the uterine lining, and secretion of the hormones). These individual processes are shown in Figures 1, 2, and 3 respectively. Although they are illustrated separately, they interact simultaneously to form a complex chain of events that occurs each month.

The series of events begins with the master controller of the cycle, the *hypothalamus*. As a vital part of the brain, it governs many functions, including appetite, weight, water balance, and moods. Should anything disturb, alter, or influence this section of the mid-brain, or any of the hormones it secretes, any or all of these functions may be affected.

The hypothalamus begins the cycle by stimulating a small endocrine gland, the *pituitary*, to secrete a hormone called the *follicle-stimulating hormone (FSH)*. As the name implies, FSH stimulates the growth of a follicle residing within one of the ovaries. As the follicle grows and the egg within it develops, it manufactures estradiol, more commonly called *estrogen*. All of these processes comprise the first half of the menstrual cycle, appropriately called the *estrogenic stage* since estrogen is the predominant hormone. Throughout this half of the cycle, the levels of estrogen increase, reaching a peak about midpoint. The rising levels of the ovarian hormone stimulate the lining of the uterus, the *endometrium*, to grow and form numerous blood vessels and glands that supply nourishment for the developing egg.

As the egg matures inside one of the follicles it slowly moves toward the periphery of the ovary. Simultaneously, the ovarian surface weakens and disintegrates, enabling the egg to burst through. As it erupts, the follicle secretes a large gush of estrogen and with it a little *progesterone*. Either the estrogen or the combination of the two hormones triggers the hypothalamus, which in turn signals the pituitary to release its hormones, LH and FSH. It is the LH or *luteinizing hormone* that predominates at this point.

With the surge of pituitary hormones, and the bursting of the egg, comes ovulation. For most women this activity happens unnoticed. For others, however, there may be some discharge from the vagina, headaches, the beginning of premenstrual symptoms, or pain. The specific cramping feeling experienced by some women at ovulation is called *"mittelschmerz"* and can actually be strong enough to be confused with appendicitis.(2)

It is often stated that ovulation occurs midpoint through the cycle. While this is correct for a 28-day cycle, it is not accurate for a 36-day cycle. A more reliable method of figuring ovulation date would be to count backward 14 days from the first day of menstruation. For instance, women with a 36-day cycle should subtract 14 from 36; therefore, they ovulated on approximately day 22. Allowing for variation, it could be from day 20 to day 24. Ovulation is not always predictable. Other factors that may affect this schedule, for example, are mental stress, physical stress, and drugs.

Once ovulation has occurred, the remnant follicle changes its structure to what is called the *corpus luteum*. The corpus luteum continues to secrete a small amount of estrogen but, more important, produces large quantities of progesterone. Because it is progesterone that is more active during this phase, the second half of the cycle is referred to as the *progestational stage*. While the endometrium has been continuously growing in the previous stage, now, under the influence of progesterone, it becomes very thick and spongy and develops many mucus-secreting glands that are capable of nourishing a fertilized egg, should fertilization occur.

If fertilization does not take place, there is no reason for nourishment, and hormone production declines. The reduction in progesterone triggers the pituitary to stop its secretion of LH. Having lost its support system, the endometrium breaks down and is sloughed off. Menstruation begins.

Mention should also be made at this time of a third pituitary hormone, *prolactin*. While once it was thought to be related only to breast development and the production of milk, more recently it has been proven to be related to the menstrual cycle. Prolactin is secreted by the pituitary gland and affects the way FSH and LH influence the ovaries and the corpus luteum. The output of prolactin increases especially at the time of ovulation and continues into the progestational stage. **Extra prolactin in the blood can upset the mechanisms controlling the production of estrogen and progesterone.**(3)

Throughout the month, the hormones are in a state of flux, rising and falling, triggering and suppressing other hor-

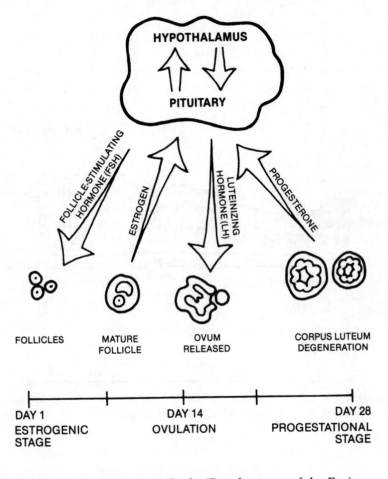

Figure 1   The Ovarian Cycle (Development of the Egg) and the Hormonal Feedback System

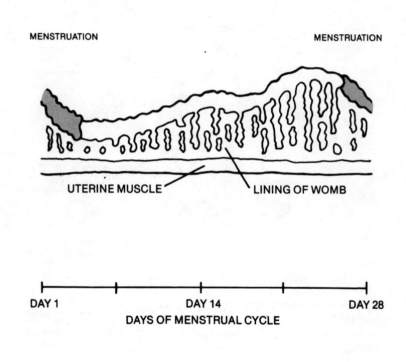

Figure 2   The Endometrial Cycle (Changes in the Uterine
Lining)

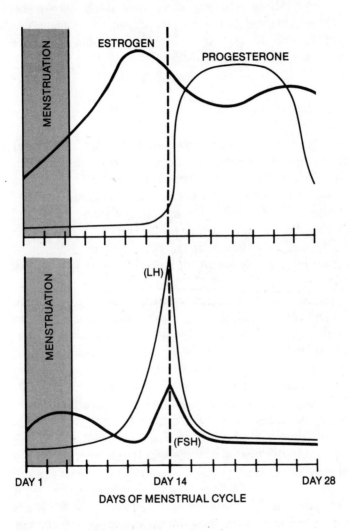

Figure 3   Monthly Hormone Levels

mones and glands. The whole feedback mechanism is extremely delicate and can be thrown off balance by many factors. If this does happen, if the body becomes out of balance for any reason, distress symptoms will occur.

Cyclic Irregularities

Both at the beginning (menarche) and at the end (menopause) of the cycle, irregularities are common. The transformations taking place in young girls approaching womanhood and the adjustments of mature women entering menopause often result in sporadic menstrual periods and in a variety of related symptoms. Because it takes time for the body to readjust to the new physiological balance, irregularity is not unusual.

Even between menarche and menopause there are times when deviations are normal. Pregnancy and lactation, for example, are welcome postponements of the monthly ritual. There are other conditions, not quite so pleasant, that can upset the cycle: a functional disorder, a genetic abnormality, being underweight or overweight, stress, and nutrient deficiency. These conditions may manifest themselves in a variety of ways in different women. They can cause irregular periods, excessive bleeding, painful periods, emotional problems, or even a cessation of the cycle. Clearly it is a complex situation; therefore when there is any major change in the normal cycle the first step women must take is to consult a competent physician.

In the majority of women there is no evidence of an organic problem. The difficulty is more likely to be the result of a chemical imbalance. It is this area to which the book is directed, to the more common menstrual problems which are caused by a hormonal imbalance and which can be corrected or at least reduced by proper nutrition and good health habits.

Menarche (The Beginning of Menstruation)

The first menstrual period marks the onset of female reproductive activity. It is usually characterized by a growth spurt in girls between the ages of ten and fifteen years; however, it has been slowly developing long before that first important day. Many bodily transformations that have been occurring gradually become obvious only just prior to puberty. It is these external manifestations that are most noticeable. The pelvic bone structure widens, and fat pads develop over the hips to give the body a fuller shape. Breasts emerge, and pubic and underarm hair begins to grow. Whether or not these changes are accepted happily depends a great deal on cultural and family attitudes.

Internal changes are much less visible. Only rarely is a girl conscious of the fact that the vaginal cavity is getting deeper, the cell walls are thickening, and the entire uterus is growing in size. Also enlarging and maturing are the ovaries, which, when they reach a certain stage of development, find themselves surrounded by numerous blood vessels. As more vascular channels emerge, the hormones from the pituitary start to impact on the female organ, resulting in the increased production of estrogen. Usually the hormonal interactions between the ovaries and the pituitary are not sufficient to cause complete development of the egg, but they can be enough to cause menstrual cycles during which partially developed eggs are formed.(4)

Eventually the amount of estrogen becomes more constant and triggers the release of the hypothalamic hormones. Until this happens, until the hypothalamus is sufficiently stimulated to secrete its hormones, menstruation will not begin. It is generally accepted that the ultimate responsibility of menarche rests in the brain, for until the hypothalamus reaches a certain level of maturity, puberty cannot commence.(5)

Once menstruation has begun, it is normally irregular for the first few years, taking three to four years before the pattern is stable. The interval between periods, the amount of flow, and the duration of bleeding may all vary considerably among girls as well as for each individual girl during this time.

In adolescents, periods can occur for some time before a mature egg is actually released from the ovary, and for this reason girls just beginning their cycles are at first relatively infertile. But this not always true, and it is conceivable that they may be ovulating and therefore could become pregnant.

Even when the cycle becomes so regular that it is predictable, many circumstances can upset it. The hypothalamus, which controls the cycle, is also instrumental in the functioning of the nervous system. Consequently, there is a relationship between the two systems, so that if one is aggravated, the other is likely to be influenced. **It is well known that stress or anxiety can alter the timing of the period and bring out symptoms of tension, depression, and cramps.** Not only emotional stress but also factors causing physical stress, such as drugs, sickness, dieting, and obesity often lead to menstrual irregularities. It is believed by some authorities that this could be a defense mechanism designed by Mother Nature to prevent a woman from becoming pregnant when there is already too much stress on her system.

Studies made in the United States and Europe indicate

that menarche has been occurring at steadily earlier ages for the past century, and continues to decline. The average age has dropped at a rate of three to four months every ten years. While the normal age in 1900 was 14.2 years, by 1975 it was down to 12.5 years. (6)   It is predicted that by the year 2000 menstruation will begin around eleven years and nine months of age. (7)

Many factors contribute to this acceleration in the growth process: diet, height, weight, cultural advantage, malfunctioning thyroid, amount of exercise, and even, believe it or not, exposure to music. Several authorities attribute early maturation to the "better nutritional standards" of the more affluent countries. However, Otto Schaeffer, M.D., who has researched this subject extensively, challenges this theory. He contends that it is in fact an inferior nutritional life-style that leads to premature menarche.

In studies done with the Canadian Eskimos, Dr. Schaeffer found that people living in countries considered primitive for their lack of technological advances enjoy near-perfect health. Upon changing their eating habits from food fresh off the land to the processed, refined foods of the more modern countries, however, they begin to develop the diseases rampant in the so-called advanced civilizations—obesity, diabetes, and heart disease. Another change he observed was that within a couple of generations on a highly refined diet, young girls begin their puberty two years earlier. (8)   Dr. Schaeffer concludes that "earlier puberty and more rapid growth are both closely linked to the epidemiologly of civilization afflications." Thus it is a poor or inadequate diet, not better nutrition, that is responsible for early menarche. It is said that some Eastern countries have known and utilized this information for years, depriving their young girls of protein in order to delay the menstrual period and the inevitable costly wedding which must take place immediately upon onset of menstruation.

Dr. Schaeffer's research suggests that diet is indeed a determining factor in early maturation. What apparently occurs in the body, he finds, is that heavy sugar consumption stimulates the hormone and endocrine system to accelerate growth and sexual development. This explanation seems plausible when one remembers that it is stimulation of these endocrine glands that does, in fact, begin the cycle.

Some gynecologists find that body weight, rather than age, is a more accurate predictor of menarche, for most girls menstruate when they reach a body weight of 92 to 101 pounds. Often this weight does coincide with the normal age of adolescents about to start puberty. When it does not, when younger girls are heavy or when older girls are extremely thin, then this fact is more clearly demonstrated.

Another factor involved in the premature puberty of some children is their reduced physical activity. Studies show that the average age of onset of menstruation for girls involved in school athletics is 13.58 years while the average for nonathletic girls is 12.23 years—more than one year's difference.(9)

Without a doubt, all the research indicates that the lifestyle of the teenage girl contributes to early menstruation. Consumption of excessive sugar, over-refined foods, childhood obesity, and lack of adequate exercise may force them to grow up at an accelerated rate. This life-style is harmful in many ways. Not only does it pave the way for poor health habits and weight problems, but it also upsets the hormonal balance and promotes emotional and physical problems. Young girls are not mentally and emotionally capable of handling a mature body, and the situations that could arise may be disastrous.

Physical problems often develop from poor living habits. **Constant hormone stimulation over the course of many years has proven to be the root of many serious disorders that plague women later on in life, the least of which may be menstrual difficulties.**

2

Menstrual Irregularities

Amenorrhea

The medical term for the absence of menstrual periods is *amenorrhea*. It is divided into two broad categories: primary amenorrhea, which is the condition of not ever having menstruated, and secondary amenorrhea, which is the cessation of menstruation in women who have previously had normal cycles. In both forms the inability to experience monthly periods is not considered an illness in itself but rather a symptom of some underlying cause. In the majority of cases, amenorrhea is the result of a hormonal imbalance.(1) Many factors can initiate this imbalance: congenital abnormalities, tumors, chronic disease, severe infection, stress, extreme weight loss and hormonal disorders. Normally the origin is not rare or unusual.

Primary amenorrhea is common in girls who do not have an adequate amount of body fat. Quite simply, they do not weigh enough for the pituitary and the hypothalamus to start releasing the hormones necessary to begin the cycle. Fat and estrogen have a close relationship, and in order for hormone production to commence, women's bodies must contain at least 17 percent fat. (2)

Lack of body fat can be the result of being underweight, or it can be caused by excessive physical activity, or by a combination of both. The intense physical exertion of gymnasts, dancers, and swimmers, for example, can impede the normal fat-to muscle ratio in the body to the degree that menstruation is delayed. It has been discovered that athletic adolescents start their periods later than the general population.

Not nearly as common, but a possibility nevertheless in postponing the cycle is obesity. In primary amenorrhea this is thought to be more of an emotional rather than a physical difficulty.

Secondary amenorrhea is usually defined as such after three periods have been missed. If the periods have not stopped because of pregnancy or menopause, the areas to investigate are low or excess body weight, overexertion, stress, and undernutrition.

Just as the body's lean-to-fat ratio is vital to begin the process of menstruation, it is also necessary to maintain it. In a study of college athletes Frische and McArthur found that when women lose ten to fifteen percent of their body weight, which represents a loss of about a third of their body fat, they become amenorrheic. (3)   Strenuous physical exercise and extreme weight loss brought on by sickness or dieting can reduce body composition sufficiently to terminate the reproductive cycle. A London research group discovered that women suffering from dietary amenorrhea have an impairment in function of the luteinizing hormone which triggers ovulation.(4)   Not having enough body fat prevents the pituitary from releasing its hormone (LH) which is necessary in signaling the cycle to begin.

Exercise can be linked to ovulation and the menstrual cycle in yet another way. According to a *Time* magazine article, during stressful workouts the body pours through the bloodstream a natural opium-like substance called *beta-endorphin*, which has been shown to suppress the female hormones that regulate menstruation.(5)   If the body is continually secreting this hormone-inhibiting chemical the results are obvious—no hormones, no period. This reaction, plus an inadequate amount of body fat, is responsible for women runners in training for a marathon not having regular periods. Once the race is over and a less arduous exercise regimen is established, their cycles return to normal.

At the opposite extreme, an excessive amount of body fat can also cause amenorrhea or irregular bleeding. Lucienne Lanson, M.D., explains how this could occur.

> Since small amounts of estrogen are normally stored in body fat, the more fatty tissue you have, the more estrogen is likely to be removed from your bloodstream and retained in these areas. Being extremely overweight also means that the body needs an increased blood plasma volume to nourish the excess adipose tissue. A larger plasma volume further dilutes the concentration of circulating estrogen.(6)

Any form of estrogen deficiency can be sufficient to disrupt the hormonal balance necessary for regular periods. Just losing the excess weight can restore normal menstruation in some women.

Secondary amenorrhea can also be psychologically induced. Many studies have conclusively shown that the brain can have a significant impact on the menstrual cycle. The effect of the higher centers of the brain on the cycle is dramatically demonstrated in a condition called *pseudocyesis*, more commonly known as false pregnancy. Women can become so convinced that they are pregnant that their periods suddenly stop. Exactly how that part of the brain that controls mood and emotion influences the hypothalamus to alter ovulation is not clearly understood. However, it is universally accepted that stresses of all kinds can modify the menstrual cycle. Changes in living conditions, such as a new job or a new home, emotional traumas like a death in the family or divorce—anything that produces tension, anxiety, and frustration can cause a temporary halt to the monthly period.

It is agreed that one of the most common causes of amenorrhea is poor health. Adelle Davis found in her research that cessation of menstrual flow and irregular menstruation are signs of widespread malnutrition. She illustrates this dramatically by relating the experiences of women who were in prisons and concentration camps during World War II and developed menstrual abnormalities. The problem (malnutrition), she states, is accompanied by a marked decrease in the production of sex hormones, and often by a shriveling of the breasts and ovaries. (7)   Cyclic regularity, intensity, and duration are mainly a function of estrogen, and the alteration of the estrogen levels brought about by a change in body size or fat composition causes periods to become irregular and even stop. When women are not nourished adequately, for whatever reason, they are subject to hormone irregularities and a variety of symptoms.

In the United States one rarely sees such an extreme situation of malnutrition. Yet there is a form of self-starvation that is becoming increasingly apparent. *Anorexia nervosa* primarily affects adolescent girls who desparately want to be thin. The physical symptoms produced as a result of extreme loss of body weight closely resemble those of the women prisoners studied by Adelle Davis. Absence of menstrual periods is just one of the many disastrous effects observed. Because the condition is both psychological and nutritional, treatment must include emotional counseling combined with a specific dietary program.

When women stop taking the oral contraceptive pill they may experience temporary amenorrhea, since it often takes time for the hormonal system to normalize itself. In their book *Women and the Crisis Sex Hormones*, Barbara Seaman and Gideon Seaman, M.D., cite countless reports of post-pill amenorrhea and infertility. While many doctors attempt to solve the problem by prescribing even more hormones, this is generally unnecessary, as most cases correct themselves within a few months to two years, and with proper nutrition in an even shorter frame of time.(8)

Menorrhagia

Menorrhagia is the medical term for profuse or excessive uterine bleeding during menstruation. It can be a symptom of infection, inflammation, polyps, or emotional difficulties. It also may be caused by something as simple as the improper placement of an intra-uterine device (IUD). Since the functional disorders are more remote possibilities, other factors will be considered here.

Excessive flow, as well as other menstrual difficulties, may indicate an underactive thyroid. It is well known that the thyroid and its hormones regulate metabolic activity. What may not be as well recognized are the widespread effects it has on other body processes and organs. As far as the reproductive cycle is concerned, the thyroid is an indispensable agent in producing the female hormones, estrogen and progesterone. The hormones of the thyroid are responsible for stimulating the pituitary, which in turn triggers the release of thyroxine, the molecule that stimulates the ovaries to produce estrogen.

It is known that a lack of adequate nutrients can decrease the effectiveness of the thyroid in regulating its various hormones. Inadequate iodine, for example, can disrupt normal functioning of the gland and lead to a buildup of estrogen. (9) Not only does a high estrogen level cause abnormal uterine bleeding, but accumulating evidence links it to chronic cystic mastitis, endometriosis, uterine fibroids, a tendency to blood clotting, and breast and uterine cancer.(10)

Good nutrition is vital in maintaining a healthy thyroid. Medical nutritionists report that hypothyroidism disappears without the use of hormones in response to an improved diet; furthermore, without an adequate diet even thyroid medication is ineffective.(11)

Excessive menstrual bleeding may be both the cause and the result of an iron deficiency anemia. While it has long been recognized that loss of blood may lead to iron deficiency anemia, it is less common to hear that a lack of the mineral will promote excessive bleeding. However, investigators at Harvard have found that iron deficiency may cause excessive menstrual bleeding by weakening the uterine muscles.(12) This phenomenon results from the great affinity hemoglobin, the substance which carries the oxygen to the cells, has for the iron that is stored in the body. When the normal supply of iron is missing, the hemoglobin may steal it from a tissue enzyme. This can result in a weakening of the uterine muscles, inadequate contractions of the blood vessels in the uterus, and heavy menstrual flow.

Problems in the hypothalamus, the pituitary glands, and the ovaries can be responsible for hormonal imbalances and abnormal bleeding. Any organ or gland in the body that is related to the production and control of hormones may be responsible. Since the kidney is needed for the elimination of estrogen from the body, a chronic kidney infection can also cause an abnormally high level of estrogen. Similarly the liver, which is involved in the degradation of estrogen to a less active and less threatening compound, if defective, can lead to an excessive estrogen supply and thus a hormonal imbalance.

Many of these situations, though certainly not all, can be corrected by nutrients alone. **Because poor nutrition is often responsible for the malfunctioning of organs, in many cases proper nutrition can revive them.**

3

Dysmenorrhea

Dysmenorrhea is a general term meaning painful menstruation. Pain, however, is not the only symptom of dysmenorrhea. Other symptoms include: backache, headache, weight-gain, constipation, diarrhea, depression, anxiety, irritability, insomnia, and a craving for sweets. Different women experience different symptoms. In a survey conducted by Paula Weideger, 24 percent of the women who responded experienced physical symptoms, 18 percent had emotional problems, and 46 percent reported both physical and psychological problems.(1)

Types of Dysmenorrhea

There are two types of dysmenorrhea: primary, indicating that the problem has no organic cause, and secondary, meaning the pain is the result of a condition such as fibroids, tumors, or endometriosis. In order to eliminate the latter possibility it is necessary to consult a gynecologist. More often than not, however, menstrual problems are not due to functional disorders, and it is the primary types of common monthly difficulties with which this book is concerned.

Doctors often categorize menstrual symptoms into two groups. The first type is called *spasmodic* and, as indicated by the name, involves spasms of acute pain localized in the inside of the thighs and lower back. These cramps, which can range from mild twinges to incapacitating spasms, normally begin on the first day of menstruation and last three to four days.

Severe cramps occur only in women who ovulate. Since it takes a few years before ovulatory patterns become established, many adolescents do not experience cramps. Women taking the contraceptive pill also may notice their cramps subside immediately upon starting the Pill. Because its function is to suppress ovulation physicians like to prescribe the Pill solely for monthly pain. Unfortunately, the associated risks prevent it from being an adequate long-term treatment.

Congestive dysmenorrhea, the second type of pain, covers an entire range of symptoms that many women experience during the period of time preceding the menstrual flow. The broad array of problems associated with the congestive type of disorder is often referred to as "Premenstrual Syndrome" (PMS), and the common symptoms are listed in Figure 4.

The manner in which women experience PMS is based on their personal body chemistries. While some women crave a candy bar others gain ten pounds and break out in pimples. Some women are fortunate enough to suffer minor aches and pains while more sorely afflicted friends pray desperately for emotional control.

Generally speaking, the premenstrual syndrome occurs after ovulation, increases until the onset of menstruation and then subsides. Women are most likely to develop the problem after 30 years of age, frequently following the birth of a baby or at the termination of the birth control pill. Strangely, neither women with hysterectomies nor menopausal women are immune to the problem.

One can best diagnose PMS by charting one's menstrual periods for a few months, particularly noticing specific combinations of symptoms that occur at the same phase of the cycle. Characteristically, the discomfort period is followed by a symptom-free period which women refer to as a time of complete euphoria.

Fortunately, PMS is now being publicly acknowledged and clinics are springing up in all the major cities in the U.S.A. Women can finally stand up and shout "I told you so!" Qualified physicians, psychologists, and nutritionists are working with women at various levels of need to help in controlling their symptoms. But the process of healing is not instantaneous. Each female is different and each one requires an individualized and integrated program.

Cause of Dysmenorrhea

At one time it was considered questionable whether the physical and emotional symptoms of dysmenorrhea were real. Women were told their pain was "all in their heads," and were given tranquilizers to calm them down. This is no longer the case—or should not be.

At last there is a physiological explanation for menstrual problems. After all these years, it has finally been proven that a chemical substance called prostaglandin is produced in excessive amounts in women with menstrual discomforts. It is this substance which apparently causes the pain as well as some of the related symptoms experienced by women with monthly problems.

Prostaglandin is an extremely powerful, hormone-like chemical that is derived from unsaturated fatty acids in the diet. It is broken down through a series of chemical reactions

Physical Aspect	Psychological Aspect
Bloating	Depression
Headaches	Anxiety
Backaches	Irritability
Joint pain	Insomnia
Breast tenderness	Irrational acts
Clumsiness	Prone to crying
Acne	Panic attacks
Cold sores	Mental confusion
Asthma	Distortion of thought perception
Allergic attacks	Uncontrollable craving for foods, especially sugar and chocolate
Epilepsy (rare)	

Figure 4   Common Symptoms of Premenstrual Syndrome

and distributed to nearly every cell of the body. A function of one type of prostaglandin (there are many kinds) is to regulate the tone of the smooth or involuntary muscles. Thus the uterine lining, being a smooth muscle, is controlled by prostaglandin. As the menstrual fluid is expelled, the uterus contracts. If too much prostaglandin is being produced the contractions become excessive and painful.

Increased prostaglandin levels also affect the amount and the activity of chemical transmitters present in the brain. Moods and emotions can be drastically altered when neurotransmitters are not operating at peak performance, and this is also part of the premenstrual syndrome.

The reason for this overproduction of prostaglandin probably lies in the cyclic variations of the hormones estrogen, progesterone, and prolactin, as well as the ratio of one hormone to another.(2)   This understanding—that it is an imbalance of the female hormones that causes monthly problems—also provides a basis on which treatment can be formulated.

Treatment with Drugs

If treating monthly symptoms were the only goal, the medical community has certainly provided several effective palliatives. For each physical and emotional symptom of dysmenorrhea there is a drug that will provide temporary relief. Of the drugs used to treat menstrual disturbances the most popular are hormones, like the oral contraceptive; pain killers and antiprostaglandins such as aspirin; and the ever-present tranquilizers. Unfortunately, these chemicals do nothing to remedy the actual problem, therefore they must be repeated month after month. Many times the continued use of the drug does more harm than the original symptom.

The Pill is not only a method of contraception, it is also a form of hormone therapy used in the treatment of painful periods. The most widely used pills contain varying amounts of synthetically produced progesterone and natural estrogen. They work by preventing ovulation. Through manipulation of the hormones the natural process of the cycle is altered and menstruation is eliminated. Many women do not realize that they have not menstruated, as there is "withdrawal bleeding" closely resembling the menstrual discharge.

Just why menstrual periods are less painful when ovulation is absent is not entirely understood. The most promising theory is that the altered hormone levels diminish the production of prostaglandin and thereby prevent cramps. Because prostaglandin is manufactured in the lining of the uterus shortly before menstruation, women who do not ovulate have only one-fifth the amount of the chemical in their menstrual fluid as do women who ovulate normally.(3)   Less prostaglandin means less pain. This is why for some women the Pill is effective in relieving pain. For others the relief is temporary, and the pain returns after a few months to a year.(4)

There is substantial evidence concerning the risks involved in hormone treatment. According to Barbara Seaman and Gideon Seaman, M.D., "to take the Pill for dysmenorrhea is a drastic measure—it's like using a cannon to kill a sparrow, and the potential price is high."(5)   Some of the minor side effects women have encountered as a result of taking the oral contraceptive are stomach cramps, nausea, headaches, breast tenderness, irregular menstrual flow, depression, acne, bleeding gums, visual disturbances, and weight gain. However, it is the more insidious effects of the

Pill to which the Seamans refer in their statement—conditions, for example, that affect the clotting characteristics of the blood and possibly promote heart attacks, strokes, and pulmonary embolisms. Reports indicate that death from the clot-forming diseases occurs about five times more frequently if one has been taking the Pill for five years or longer.(6)

The oral contraceptive has also repeatedly been linked to cancer. Dr. Otto Saratorius, Director of the Cancer Control Clinic of Santa Barbara General Hospital in California, reports that:

> After a two year study of two hundred young women, there are indications that a majority of those women who used the Pill for birth control are sustaining irreversible and permanent breast damage, and are exposing themselves to an approximate three-fold increase in the risk of developing breast cancer—the direct result of overstimulation of the breast by estrogen and progesterone.(7)

Estrogen turns nutrition into a state of chaos by depleting vitamin and mineral supplies and upsetting the nutrient balance. Just as it is necessary to have the complete spectrum of nutrients for optimum health, it is vital to body functioning and equilibrium to receive these nutrients in definite proportions and ratios. For this reason, use of the Pill involves a dangerous risk. Dr. Harold Speert, a Columbia University gynecologist known for his contribution to endocrinology, sums it up:

> There is almost no organ or tissue which if studied has not been shown to be affected by the Pill to some degree.

>The Pill acts through the pituitary gland, "the master gland" and even "the conductor of the endocrine symphony." It does a lot of important things which shouldn't be interfered with. It's unrealistic to think that long-range effects will not be inevitable.(8)

Various other drugs are commonly recommended in alleviating the symptoms of dysmenorrhea. They can be as mild as aspirin or as powerful as codeine. Aspirin is both an analgesic, or pain reliever, and a mild prostaglandin inhibitor. It is taken either alone or as a primary ingredient in many over-the-counter medications like Midol and Pamprin. The drug is so easily available that people underestimate its potential for toxicity if improperly used. While it is relatively safe, aspirin is not totally harmless, and the Food and Drug Administration has warned that many of its side-effects can be serious, especially for certain groups. These include pregnant women, people with bleeding disorders, and people taking other drugs or alcohol. Possible side-effects include heartburn, stomach discomfort, nausea, vomiting, stomach ulcers, bleeding from the lining of the stomach, and gastrointestinal hemorrhage.(9)

For women with severe menstrual discomfort aspirin is only partially effective; therefore, the stronger antiprostaglandins are normally prescribed. These include Motrin, Indocin, or Ponstel. Because the drug has to be more potent to be effective, it stands to reason that the potential side-effects must also be greater. Motrin, representative of these drugs, has the following reactions: gastric upset, peptic ulcers, nausea, heartburn, anemia, abdominal pain, diarrhea, vomiting, dizziness, skin rash, itching, blurred vision and cataracts.(10)

The use of tranquilizers such as Valium and Librium remains a common practice in treating menstrual disorders. In spite of the overwhelming information on the chemical basis of dysmenorrhea, many doctors still consider the premenstrual syndrome as primarily a psychological problem. This is evidenced by the number of prescriptions written for Valium alone—more than 75 million per year, with more than two-thirds of these prescribed for women.(11)

While the manufacturers and medical practitioners have touted Valium and other mood-altering drugs as highly effective, there are consequences of taking them that cannot be overlooked. Valium anesthetizes the emotions, dulls the brain, clouds the thinking process, and slows down reflexes. It sedates the senses and can cause depression. It is also addictive, capable of producing both a psychological and a physical dependence. The addiction problem is so serious that it is now estimated that over two million women in this country are medicated "junkies" who cannot get through the day without their pills.(12)

Drug Therapy Versus Vitamin Therapy

Most drugs are palliative—they alleviate symptoms but do nothing to cure or restore the body to its healthful state. In fact, many drugs actually promote more problems than they relieve. Statistics show that every year up to 150,000 people die from overprescription.

Why then do physicians prescribe pills so freely, if it is known that the chemicals are harmful and there is an alternative? The problem is two-fold. The first difficulty seems to be in the doctors' lack of training in the area of clinical nutrition.

Orthodox medical schools emphasize the diagnosis and treatment of disease through drugs. Little attention is directed at alternative health practices and even less time is given to the prevention of disease. One cannot blame the doctor for his or her educational bias or lack of knowledge in the area of nutrition. The field of medicine is too broad for any one person or group of persons to master.

The other side of the story concerns the individual. Too often people demand an instant cure from the health care professional, rather than change the life-style that is promoting their weakened condition. Some people prefer masking symptoms to giving up a favorite habit even though it is harmful. So it is not entirely the physician who is to blame. Ultimately, the responsibility for personal health care rests with the individual. People, therefore, need to be informed as to how their body functions, what causes sickness and disease, and how they can actively participate in the self-healing process.

As the scientific evidence in the field of nutrition becomes more widely accepted, increasing numbers of doctors are learning and applying this information. The fact that vitamin therapy is safer than drug therapy has long been acknowledged by the medical profession, and now research has progressed to the point where nutrients have been shown to be as effective as drugs in the treatment of many disorders.

Certainly not all drugs are harmful and to be shunned. There are times when they are necessary—even vital. But it should be remembered that a drug is a substance that is foreign to the body, and it should be taken only when required and for as short a time as possible.

Nutrients, on the other hand, are not dangerous. They are the natural, organic substances needed for maintaining life. When used in the treatment of various problems, nutrients (vitamins, minerals, and amino acids) work to establish the correct balance in the body. In doing so they can minimize temporary discomforts, provide nourishment for the entire body, and achieve long-term good health. Dr. Roger Williams, biochemist and respected authority in the field of nutrition, calls nutrients "Nature's own biological weapons," and feels they should be given top priority in the treatment of disease.(13)

Natural healing is not a new approach to treating disease. The ancient philosophers taught that if we follow the laws of Nature, the body will eventually heal itself. In the twelfth century Maimonides proclaimed: "Let nothing which can be treated by diet be treated by other means." And Hippocrates, father of all physicians, believed that drugs should be left in the chemist's pot "if thou can heal the patient with food." There are no miracles or magic elixirs, much as one would like to hope, but Nature, given its raw materials and time, will heal.

Henry Beiler, M.D., after fifty years of practice, found a direct relationship between eating improper foods and disease. In his book *Food Is Your Best Medicine* he stressed the invaluable ancient healing principles. According to Dr. Beiler "the greatest physicians have used the fewest and simplest of drugs because they were fully aware of the role of Nature in health; they knew that all the forces of Nature in man, beast, and the plant world are dedicated to obtaining and keeping a perfect state of health."(14)

In summary then: to put harmful foods and chemicals into the human body results in disease; by eliminating them, and through proper nourishment, the body can be restored to its naturally healthful state. Taking drugs is sometimes unavoidable, but if there is an alternative that is safe as well as effective, it is only logical to choose that which will "first do no harm."

The chart on the following page (Figure 5) illustrates the major differences in the ways that drugs and vitamins react in the body.

Drugs	Vitamins
Rapid in action.	Slow to take effect. May take weeks or months.
Many have a narrow and specific effectiveness.	Systemic in action. Tendency to influence the whole body.
Most effective when given alone, so their powerful biochemical agents cannot interfere with function.	Work best in combination.
Foreign, alien substances, even toxic. May cause malnutrition. 1. Depress appetite (diet pills). 2. Impair body's ability to absorb nutrients. 3. Cause loss of vitamins and minerals. 4. Interfere with mechanism for using vitamins.	Natural to body: vitamins are food. Normally found in body. Vitamins A and D toxicity is exaggerated; must be used to excess for a long period of time. On rare occasions, vitamins B and C can produce minor symptoms of distress when taken in large quantities. These are usually only slight digestive effects.

Dr. Harold Rosenberg and A. N. Feldzamen, *The Doctor's Book of Vitamin Therapy* (New York: G.P. Putnam's Sons, 1974).

Figure 5   Drugs Versus Vitamins

4

The Nutritional Approach

It has been scientifically and empirically proven that most menstrual difficulties are due to improper metabolism of the female hormones. The menstrual system is a delicate balance of hormones, glands, and organs, all of which depend on each other to function smoothly. When one part does not operate as it should, the entire equilibrium is upset. The resulting imbalance in the ratio of hormones can lead to excessive estrogen activity, increased prostaglandin production, pain, and all the symptoms associated with the premenstrual syndrome. **If the imbalance is not corrected, more serious problems can develop.**

There has been much speculation as to the original cause of hormone deficiency and excess. H. L. Newbold, M.D., a practicing psychiatrist, and other researchers have found a strong correlation between hormone inadequacy and vitamin and mineral deficiencies; furthermore, when the nutritional deficiency is corrected by diet and/or supplements, the glands often normalize.(1) A lack of adequate nutrients can actually inhibit the production of hormones creating a deficiency that ultimately results in disequilibrium and pain. To restore balance requires the correct combination of nutrients, which in some cases can exceed the minimum ranges determined by the government. Body homeostasis can be accomplished through nutrition. The human body is a marvelous mechanism, and given the right environment, it is capable of repairing itself. However, if even one nutrient is missing, sickness can develop.

When women experience menstrual problems regularly, it is most likely that they are not receiving adequate nourishment. The fact that women generally are short on even the minimum daily requirements of essential nutrients was dramatically shown in a nationwide food consumption survey prepared by the government. (See Figure 6) This study provides an explanation for the prevalence of menstrual problems, and points up the obvious relationship between poor nutrition and monthly difficulties.

It does not seem possible that American women are undernourished when food is so plentiful, yet they are. The reasons for this incongruity are many. First, availability does not necessarily ensure consumption. We may have a variety of foods to select from, but in the real world of career women, working mothers and active homemakers, the time to plan and eat quality meals is limited. Women of the eighties are often willing to settle for a quick cup of coffee and a cookie before dashing off to the next important event. Also, women's perennial obsession with dieting and maintaining a slim figure often takes precedence over nutritional judgment. Let's face it, thin is in!

Another disturbing fact that partly accounts for individuals not receiving the minimum nutritional requirements is that the food itself is not of the quality we so casually take for granted. Before food even reaches the supermarket much has

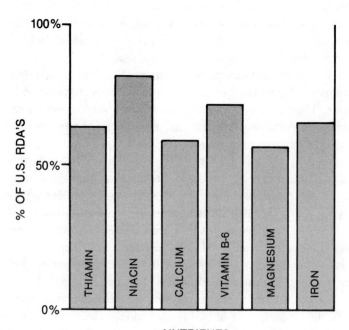

U.S.D.A. *1980 Nationwide Food Consumption Survey*

U.S. RDAs (Recommended Daily Allowances) are nutritional labeling standards determined by the United States Government based on the minimum nutrients required by individuals on a daily basis to maintain health.

Figure 6   How Do Women Stack Up Against the U.S. RDAs?

been done to it which depletes it of its life-giving nutrients. Fruits and vegetables have been sprayed in the fields with herbicides and insecticides, picked green, and ripened artificially with chemicals. They are often stored for months, transported long distances, and made presentable for display with waxes and preservatives. Grains are commonly refined beyond recognition, and filled with tongue-twisting additives. By the time the food reaches the dinner table, it has lost an estimated 50 percent of its nutrients. The remainder of the vitamins and minerals we ourselves destroy in preparation.

There are other sources of nutritional deficiencies, because the process of nutrition just begins with the consumption of food. Everything that biochemically happens to food must be considered: how it is digested, absorbed, and utilized by the body. A full study takes into consideration individual genetic weaknesses, specific body types, life styles, and external influences such as air pollution, drugs, and stress. One can see the complexity of the situation. For this reason it cannot be emphasized enough that nutritional requirements are highly individualistic. What may constitute an adequate diet for one person may be totally insufficient for another. There are too many variables to standardize one program for all. It is imperative that women examine their own weaknesses, life styles, and the specific external factors that could affect their personal nutritional requirements.

Biochemical Individuality

Nutritional requirements are as distinct as fingerprints. All women are unique unto themselves. From the length of their hair to the shape of their thighs, diversities abound. One need only go to the nearest spa and look at the ladies in their leotards and tights to see the external variety. As they perform their aerobic exercises, another distinction can be seen—how different body machines move and handle physical stress. Some women dance gracefully through the workout and barely elevate their pulse, while others breathe heavily and tire quickly. Conditioning certainly plays a role in these differences, but basic body constitution is as strong a determinant.

Internally, the human body is just as unique. The size and weight of organs and glands vary as widely as external structure. The weight of the liver, for example, varies sevenfold. The thyroid gland can weigh from eight to fifty grams, and the ovaries from two to ten grams. Since the size of the female sex glands varies, it seems logical that the amount of hormones they produce would also be different. This is true. The amount of estrogen women produce can vary by a factor of at least nine.

There is mounting evidence that a period of malnutrition can cause a permanent enzyme change within the body. Individuals who are temporarily deprived of adequate nourishment require a greater amount of some vitamins for the rest of their lives. The most dramatic illustration of this phenomenon occurred in prisoners of war who were forced to survive on severely inadequate diets. When these malnourished individuals returned to society and normal eating, they were not able to maintain their health without the aid of specific nutrients. This, of course, is an extreme condition which does not occur in everyday living. And then again, maybe it does, though perhaps on a smaller scale. Consider the young women who diet to the point of malnutrition, or the junk-food junkies who live solely on french fries, cokes, and cookies. They are not totally without food, as was the prisoner of war, nevertheless they too are undernourished. And while they may feel fine for many years, especially if they are young, there will come a day when the body simply will not handle it anymore. The elaborate system of chemical responses that has been compensating for years will no longer be able to cope. When essential nutrients are missing for an extended period of time, weaknesses of one form or another will develop, and these can manifest themselves in menstrual problems or find other forms of expression.

The Changed American Diet

Within the last forty years the average American diet has changed drastically. While people once enjoyed home-cooked meals made from locally grown fruit and vegetables, today they rely on fast-food restaurants, instant dinners, frozen entrées, canned vegetables and packaged sweets for their nourishment. Convenience has taken over. In 1940 processed foods represented 10 percent of the American diet; in 1970 they made up about 50 percent. Now, a decade later, they comprise about 60 percent of the daily intake.

Food processing technology has completely changed the eating habits of the people of this nation. Complex carbohydrates have been replaced by simple sugars, and dietary fiber has decreased while the consumption of fat has increased. These substitutions have been a serious detriment to the health of our society, and have promoted numerous diseases that are rampant in the United States today.

The most obvious shift in the American way of eating is the move from a predominantly complex carbohydrate diet

to a simple carbohydrate diet. Government studies show that the reduction in complex carbohydrates is. approximately 54 percent, paralleled by a 50 percent increase in simple sugars. People are eating fewer whole-grain products, fresh fruit and vegetables, and are substituting white flour-based breads and cereals and refined sugars as found in cakes, cookies, crackers, and soda pop. Dr. Robert Atkins, a specialist in nutritional medicine, believes "this huge jump in sugar consumption is probably the most drastic dietary change man has made in his whole fifty million years of existence."(2)

Sugar and other highly refined carbohydrates are poor food choices for many reasons. In terms of nutrient content, they add little if anything at all to the body. More importantly, in order to be metabolized they actually drain the body of other vitamins and minerals, especially the B vitamins. All carbohydrates require a certain amount of B-Complex vitamins in order to be utilized by the body. Without them the carbohydrates, or fuel foods, cannot burn properly. Natural complex carbohydrates such as whole grain products, fruits and vegetables are richly supplied with the necessary nutrients for metabolisation. Processed and refined flours, cereals, rice, and sugar are not. Unburned carbohydrates, which are the simple sugars lacking the essential vitamins needed to metabolize them, produce nervousness, indigestion, constipation, and any number of disorders. The Senate Select Committee on Nutrition recommend in their "Dietary Goals" that Americans reduce their sugar consumption by 40 percent and increase their consumption of complex carbohydrates from about 28 percent of energy intake to about 48 percent.(3)   This change alone could reduce numerous problems and symptoms.

Consumption of fats has also increased tremendously during the past fifty years. Fats now account for approximately 40 percent of the calories in an average daily diet. While the human body does need a certain amount of fat to provide fuel, help utilize the fat-soluble vitamins, and protect the nerves, excess amounts have been linked to cardiovascular disease, high blood pressure, diabetes, liver and gall bladder disorders, obesity, and even breast cancer. Dr. Ernst L. Wynder, President and Medical Director of the American Health Foundation in New York, testified before a Senate Committee that "Breast cancer, the biggest killer of all cancers in women, is associated worldwide with the consumption of a high fat diet."(4)

The United States Department of Agriculture (U.S.D.A.) has divided fats into two groups. The first are the easily recognizable, visible fats—butter, margarine, vegetable oils, animal fats. A variety of "hidden fats" comprise the second group, and these are found in foods like cakes, cookies, chocolate, nuts, cheese, and luncheon meats. It is this group which we must become aware—and wary—of. The U.S.D.A. estimates that approximately 60 percent of all the fat Americans consume is in this invisible category. The suggestion of the Senate Committee is to reduce all fats from the current average of 40 percent to 30 percent of total energy output. Many nutritionists recommend cutting that number further to 20 percent.

As sugar and fat have increased in the diet, dietary fiber has decreased. Various studies indicate that the incidence of heart attack, cancer of the colon, diverticulosis, and many other problems increases in direct proportion to the decrease in the amount of roughage. This loss of fiber has occurred as a result of the refining and processing of whole grains and cereals. For reasons of economics and distribution, the food industry has processed virtually all of the natural nutrients out of the most frequently consumed foods. Whole grain breads have been stripped of their bran and wheat, which contain not only the fiber but also the vitamins and minerals. Rice, cereals, and pastas have been reduced to nothing but carbohydrates. True, manufacturers have enriched the various grains with a few token vitamins, but not nearly in the quantities they have destroyed.

The nominal addition of the standard six nutrients is not only a meager attempt at revitalizing products, it is also a corruption of the mysterious laws of Nature. Food in its original form is perfectly balanced. The nutrients within the food are proportioned according to a specific ratio and work together harmoniously and synergistically within the cells of the body. Unknown vitamins and minerals exist, as well as the named ones, and they work together in digesting and utilizing the food in a most efficient manner. When men alter Nature's perfect formula by removing some ingredients and adding others, the balance is distorted. The U.S. government publicly acknowledges this principle:

> In bread, as with other foods undergoing processing, there is the danger that, as the degree of processing increases, nutrients known and unknown are removed or altered in ways not currently understood. (6)

To eat foods as close to nature as possible is most important for good health.

Technically the word fiber refers to all those components

of food that cannot be broken down by enzymes in the human digestive tract. It is the undigested portion of the plant product, in fact, that makes it so beneficial. Fiber is able to pass quickly through the colon, reducing the amount of time harmful waste materials might linger and accumulate. The faster our food passes through the digestive tract the better, for when it accumulates, toxins are produced and can be reabsorbed into the body. Many conditions are known to result from a low fiber diet, constipation, hemorrhoids, and varicose veins to name a few.

To change a lifetime of eating habits takes a concerted effort on the part of those who wish to be healthy. It means eliminating "convenience" items containing refined flour and sugar, and substituting whole-grain products, fresh fruits and raw or barely cooked vegetables.

Another dramatic change in the American diet in the past few decades is the increasing number of additives introduced into the food supply. It is currently estimated that some 4,000 food additives are used regularly in the United States. Few, if any, of these chemicals have nutritional value; many are unnecessary, and some are dangerous. The White House Conference on Food, Nutrition, and Health Food Safety admitted that: "It is not possible to determine with absolute certainty the safety of the ever-increasing number of chemicals added to, or present in, our foods."(7)   The situation becomes even more alarming when one considers the possible effects of the combinations of these chemical ingredients. Latest available information indicates that the average American now ingests more than five pounds of additives per year, and so it would seem especially important to limit the amount of additives and preservatives we consume.

Need for Supplementation

Current developments in the field of nutrition have shown that vitamin and mineral supplements are much more important than was once commonly believed, and that the body requires greater quantities than previously realized. There are always the fortunate few who will live a long, healthy life without the need for supplements. A far greater majority, however, not only requires them, but often cannot enjoy a healthy life-style without them.

Dr. Roger Williams, who is probably responsible for more original work in the field of vitamin research than any other living scientist, states his belief in the value of supplementation:

> The most basic weapons in the fight against disease are those most ignored by modern medicine: the numerous nutrients that the cells of our bodies need. If our bodies are ailing—as they must be in disease—the chances are excellent that it is because they are being inadequately provisioned.(8)

Dr. E. Cheraskin and W. M. Ringsdorf, Jr., too, have currently been making nutritional history. They concur that "it is unlikely that an individual's nutrient needs or requirements can be achieved by food alone. For this reason, they suggest many other nutrients should be taken in excess of the average need as insurance against possible deficiencies."(9)

When one considers all the antagonists out to destroy the body's nutrient supply, taking supplements seems logical. Chemicals, drugs, pollution, additives, insecticides, cooking, canning, freezing, smoking, alcohol, coffee, tea, sugar, sickness, and age are among the factors that can deplete the nutrient reserves and render them unable to act.

Antagonists work in many ways. First, they may destroy the vitamin directly. For example, chlorinated water completely destroys vitamin E in the body. Smoking depletes vitamin C at the rate of about 25 mg per cigarette. And alcohol, heat, and sugar use up vitamin B reserves.

Second, an antagonist may alter the composition of the nutrient in a way that prohibits it from being used by the body. It may interfere with the conversion of a vitamin to its active coenzyme form. Mineral oil, for instance, will prevent carotene, the percursor of vitamin A, from being converted to the usable vitamin A. The antagonist may also impair the absorption and utilization of a vitamin. Chemicals in coffee and tea inhibit the absorption of iron. Birth control pills interfere with the metabolizing of vitamins B-12, B-6, and folic acid.

Finally, these nutrient enemies may cause excessive elimination of a nutrient. Drugs are especially active in this respect. Diuretics excrete not only fluid from the body but also sodium, potassium, magnesium, and B vitamins. Aspirin, even in small amounts, can triple the excretion rate of vitamin C.

The fact that vitamin and mineral supplementation is vital for optimum health is not disputed by nutritionists. The amounts required to achieve this level of well-being are another matter. Generally speaking, for those who would like to begin a basic supplement program—one that is adequate without being excessive—the advice of Professor Roslyn Alfin-Slater of the University of California at Los Angeles might be beneficial. This cautious authority has advised his medical students that a person can consume twice the RDA of fat soluble vitamins and five times the RDA of water soluble vitamins without danger of toxicity. Specific amounts that have helped large groups of women in the treatment of menstrual problems will be discussed in following chapters.

5

Nutritional Treatment of the Premenstrual Syndrome

Dysmenorrhea has often been divided into two separate categories: the Premenstrual Syndrome, and Menstrual Distress or menstrual cramps. Believing that each type originated from a different source, many doctors treated them separately. More recently, however, the literature increasingly suggests that there is one basic underlying problem which manifests itself as different symptoms in different women. **The imbalance of one or several hormones results in an overproduction of prostaglandin, and it is this substance that is primarily responsible for the numerous discomforts women experience.**

Determining where the premenstrual syndrome ends and menstrual cramps begin is not easy. While this book treats the symptoms of dysmenorrhea in separate chapters, keep in mind that the two problems often overlap.

The ultimate goal in treating individual symptoms is to achieve that ideal physiological balance that the body requires for optimum health. By accomplishing this goal present discomforts can be minimized, if not totally eliminated, and future problems may be avoided. The nutrients commonly deficient in women with menstrual problems will be discussed. While every vitamin and mineral is not listed, it must be stressed that the body functions as a unit and all nutrients are vital for good health.

The concept that nutrition and menstrual difficulties are related is not new. About twenty years ago, the internationally known nutritionist Dr. Carlton Fredericks researched the relationship between diet and menstrual problems. Believing that the symptoms could be relieved through proper nutrition, he enlisted the aid of some two hundred female students to test his theory. The results of the experiment showed that those students who improved their diets in accordance with the specifications experienced a reduction in premenstrual tension, water retention, nervousness, irritability, backaches, pains in the thighs, and sensitivity of the breasts. A majority of the women also reported a shortening of the menstrual period from the "normal" five days to three.(1)

From these studies of over two decades ago, Dr. Fredericks concluded that the basic cause of most menstrual problems was excessive estrogen activity. This earlier theory concurs with more recent discoveries that menstrual pain is definitely the result of a hormonal imbalance. Researchers disagree as to whether it is too much estrogen, too little progesterone, an imbalance in the relation between the two, or even too little prolactin that is the culprit. But what they do agree on is that it results in an imbalance in the ratio of female hormones. Normalizing the hormones—reducing those that are in excess and increasing those that are deficient—should relieve the problem and ease the pain.

Dr. Fredericks' approach specifically centered on regulating estrogen activity. To accomplish this he focused his program on the liver, where control of estrogenic activity takes place. While in the liver estrogen undergoes a degradation process. It changes from estrogen to estradiol, to estrone, and finally to its less active and less threatening form, estriol. The ability of the liver to make this conversion depends directly on its healthiness. If it is well-nourished it will break down the hormone, but if the liver is nutrient deficient it will not. When the organ fails to function as it should a hormone imbalance is created, and menstrual discomfort results.

The dietary program that Dr. Fredericks found so successful in reducing menstrual problems was based on the theory that a healthy liver would regulate estrogen activity. To achieve this he advised the women to increase their intake of the B-Complex vitamins, increase the intake of protein (if it was necessary), and reduce the amount of sugar in the diet. Each of these points, as well as other treatments found effective by various doctors and researchers, are discussed in detail below.

B-Complex Vitamins

The B-Complex vitamins are vital to the liver in the conversion of estrogen to estriol. Tests in the early 1930's proved that the flow of estrogen through the liver could be turned on or off by feeding or withholding the B vitamins in the diet.(2)   Even a severely degenerated liver, one showing extensive destruction of cells and infiltration of fat, is effective in degrading estrogen if the diet is adequate.

Not only does a vitamin B deficiency create a high level of estrogen, but an oversupply of estrogen will cause a vitamin B deficiency. One problem aggravates the other and promotes an even greater imbalance. Women taking the Pill show a significant lack of certain vitamins and minerals, especially those of the B-Complex group. (3)

An inadequate supply of B vitamins in the diet over an extended period of time can lead to problems more serious than menstrual distress. Many studies have indicated that there is a definite relationship between low amounts of B vitamins, excessive estrogen activity and estrogen-based cancers. One such study, performed at McGill Medical School, involved two groups of women, matched in age. One group suffered from uterine cancer and the other group was healthy. The results speak for themselves.

> A very large majority of the cancer patients displayed high levels of estrogen, low intake of vitamin B, and low blood levels of the vitamin. By coincidence, exactly the same percentage (94.5%) of the healthy patients had a high intake of vitamin B, high blood levels (of the vitamin), and normal or low levels of estrogen. (4)

When estrogen is not broken down it tends to lodge itself in the estrogen receptors of the breast and uterus increasing the risk of estrogen-based cancers. On the other hand, if it is reduced to estriol not only does it not promote cancer, it actually protects against it. (5)   While similar to the estrogen molecule in that it has some action as a female hormone, estriol is less active and therefore less harmful. **Making certain that the B-Complex vitamins are plentiful in the diet will not only reduce monthly pain, more importantly it may even prevent cancer of the breast and uterus.**

Vitamin B deficiency is common in America today. As the nutrients have been processed out of the whole grains, they are almost nonexistent in bread, cereal, rice, and packaged products. They are also water soluble, and therefore may be lost in cooking and heating. Other factors also increase the need for B-Complex: excessive sugar consumption, alcohol intake, stress, and drugs. Even if this group of vitamins were not needed to treat and prevent menstrual problems, they are vital for all-around good health.

There are some B vitamins that are especially useful in controlling the activity of estrogen and other hormones. These are choline, inositol, lecithin, vitamins B-6 and B-12. The first three vitamins are known as *lipotropics*, because they prevent abnormal or excessive accumulation of fat in the liver. If fatty deposits are formed around it the liver will not deactivate those hormones that are no longer useful to the body. Again, the result is hormone accumulation and imbalance.

Each of these nutrients has a variety of functions, but inositol specifically has a supplementary role in the treatment of some of the psychological symptoms characteristic of monthly distress. The literature shows this relatively unknown vitamin to have a mild anti-anxiety effect similar to that of a tranquilizer, and it can provide a viable alternative to the overprescribed Valium.

The lipotropics enable the liver to produce lecithin, an unsaturated fatty compound. Like choline and inositol, lecithin slows down the accumulation of fat in the liver by aiding in the transportation of fats and helping the cells to remove fats and cholesterol from the body. Lecithin helps to cleanse the liver and purify the kidneys. It is also a structural material for every cell in the body, particularly those of the brain, nerves, and glands, and most specifically the sex glands and the pituitary.

Lecithin is a rich source of a variety of food elements. It contains choline, inositol, and vitamins E, D, and K. It is equally rich in the essential fatty acids needed to transport the fat-soluble vitamins. When the body is supplied with untreated foods such as egg yolk, yeast, wheat germ, organ meats, and leafy green vegetables, lecithin is manufactured naturally. Without an adequate supply of these sources, the liver will not make lecithin and supplementation is necessary.

Soybean-based lecithin is found in powders, granules, and capsules. One tablespoon of the granules, or six capsules, contains 244 mg each of inositol and choline. Daily doses range from 100 mg to 500 mg. When adding extra lecithin to the diet, Earl Mindell, author of *The Vitamin Bible*, suggests adding extra calcium (calcium lactate or a chelated calcium) to keep the phosphorus and calcium in balance, as choline increases the body's need for phosphorus.

Of all the B-Complex vitamins, probably the most widely beneficial is vitamin B-6 (pyridoxine). It affects the mind, heart, skin, nervous system, stomach, kidneys, and immune system. For women its primary importance lies in the regulation, production, and utilization of estrogen.

A double-blind study conducted by Guy Abraham, M.D., former professor of obstetrics, gynecology, and endocrinology at UCLA, and Tennessee physician Joel Hargrove, M.D., showed that premenstrual tension was substantially reduced in women taking the vitamin. According to Dr. Abraham "This is a very significant finding when compared to any drug that has been tested."(6)

A deficiency of pyridoxine can be related to premenstrual tension and depression. A lack of vitamin B-6 seems to have a harmful effect on the chemical pathways in the hypothalamus and also on the pathways that connect it to the pituitary gland. The result is an imbalance in the production of dopamine and serotonin, chemicals needed to calm the nervous system.

Medical journals such as the *Lancet* have reported that vitamin B-6 can relieve the depression associated with estrogen-based contraceptives. (7)   Another study testing the effectiveness of vitamin B-6 in depression showed that considerable improvement or complete recovery occurred in 76% of women taking the vitamin, and that the participants noticed benefits within one day of administration. (8)

High estrogen levels, which occur just prior to menstruation, cause the body to retain fluids. For many years water retention within the brain tissue has been known to cause tension, headaches, depression, and premenstrual discomfort. Vitamin B-6 is extremely effective as a natural diuretic. The amount needed varies in different women, but the doses most often recommended range between 25 mg and 200 mg during the premenstrual week and as necessary thereafter.

Some doctors have had remarkable success relieving premenstrual headaches with vitamin B-6. One of the first to use pyridoxine for this purpose was Professor P. Giles of Perth, Australia. At a hospital in London over 80% of women with premenstrual headaches were completely cured, and nearly 65% of women suffering from premenstrual tension in general were either completely cured or very much improved. (9)

Menstruation-related acne has also been helped and sometimes completely alleviated by vitamin B-6. While the acne may not be altogether eliminated in all cases, nearly three out of four women report a significant reduction. (10)   Again, the dosage varies with the individual, but the amount could be as high as 400 mg per day.

The benefits of vitamin B-6 could—and do—fill volumes.

It is actually more than one vitamin, being a complex of the substances pyridoxine, pyridoxinal and pyridoxamine, which are all closely realted. Just one form, pyridoxine, is used in more than 60 enzyme systems within the body.

The rate at which people age is dependent on the ability of the cells to reproduce. Because vitamin B-6 is vital to the production of the nucleic acids, DNA and RNA, regeneration of new cells cannot take place without an adequate supply. The fact that women have a greater requirement for B-6 and are likely to be deficient may be a reason why women show their age so much more quickly than men.

Although the vitamin is widely distributed among plant and animal foods, a large percentage is lost in refining and cooking. Dr. Fredericks has revealed that "the vitamin B-6 content of the foods that comprise half our diet has been reduced to about 80%."(11)

Due to biochemical individuality, therapeutic doses could range from 5 mg to 1,000 mg. To begin with, though, Dr. Abraham recommends that women with severe premenstrual tension take 500 mg a day, and preferably in a timed-release tablet.(12)   This should be taken with a regular B-Complex supplement and other nutrients to ensure a solid nutritional foundation. Anyone taking more than 50 mg daily should also take equal amounts of vitamins B-1 and B-2 to maintain a proper balance. Dr. Michael Lesser suggests additionally taking 2,000 mg of magnesium or a chelate equivalent to 400 mg of elemental magnesium.(13)   Zinc sulfate (80 mg) is another complement of vitamin B-6 and should be taken with it.

Dr. Carl C. Pfeiffer of the Brain Bio Center uses dream recall as a yardstick to measure vitamin B-6 deficiency. People who report they do not dream or cannot remember their dreams are able to dream normally with sufficient B-6 and zinc.(14)   If the dosage is too much, sleep becomes restless, and dreams are too vivid. Reduction in the amount will solve the problem immediately.

Depression, fatigue, loss of appetite, and irritability— symptoms descriptive of "the blahs" during menstruation— have been known to occur in people with a vitamin B-12 deficiency. Even though a classical deficiency is not normally indicated, when the vitamin has been restored there is generally a feeling of well-being. In a double-blind study reported in the *British Journal of Nutrition,* a small controlled trial was carried out to investigate the theory that B-12 improved the general well-being of patients. While none of the individuals had any evidence of a physical deficiency, the results indicated a statistically significant improvement in the mood and feelings of those tested.(15)

Vitamin B-12 deficiency should be of concern to two groups in particular. First, women who take the oral contraceptive run the risk of being in short supply. According to statistics, half of the users of the Pill have B-12 levels below the normal range, and 15% are strikingly deficient. Second, vegetarians who exclude totally animal proteins such as meat, milk, eggs, cheese, or fish from their diets for five years or longer often develop sore mouths and tongues, menstrual disturbances, and a variety of nervous symptoms.(16)   In a study of women vegetarians it was reported that amenorrhea and menstrual disturbances were encountered in 8 of the 22 women tested.(17)

The best sources of vitamin B-12 are liver, dried brewers yeast, and supplements. Because it requires a specific gastrointestinal tract secretion for its absorption, B-12 is not absorbed well. Daily doses of 3 mcg to 6 mcg are sufficient for most people; however, some people have said they have much more energy and even a healthier looking skin if the supplements are more potent—from 25 mcg to 100 mcg. Vitamin B-12 is most effective when taken with folic acid.

Protein

The second recommendation Dr. Fredericks makes to control estrogenic activity is to ensure an adequate supply of protein in the diet. Protein is vital for a healthy liver and, more importantly, it is an indispensable nutrient for the entire body. Without protein the body would not grow properly or even maintain itself. Its priority in human nutrition is exemplified in the name itself, which means "of first importance."

Protein, which yields amino acids, is one of the most complex organic compounds found in Nature. Other than water, it is the most abundant component in the body. Protein is the fundamental structural element within every cell and performs several structural functions. It regulates metabolic processes and provides a source of heat and energy. Only protein can repair worn-out tissue and build new tissue—something neither fats nor carbohydrates can do. Hormones which control internal processes are protein. Enzymes that promote thousands of chemical reactions are protein. Even hemoglobin, the critical oxygen-carrying molecule of the blood, is built from protein.

In order to be utilized by the body cells, protein must be broken down into various combinations of amino acids. There are over 20 amino acids; 8 are classified as essential, and the remainder are nonessential. The difference between the two is that essential amino acids must be derived from outside sources—food—while nonessential amino acids can be synthesized from the others by the body. However, this synthesis can occur only if the amino acids are present in sufficient quantities and in the right proportions.

Proteins that contain all 8 essential amino acids are called complete proteins and are usually acquired from animal sources such as meat, fish, poultry, eggs, and milk. Proteins which contain only some of the amino acids or an insufficient quantity of a particular amino acid are labeled incomplete, and cannot maintain the body by themselves. Plant proteins which are incomplete in themselves are found in vegetables, grains, nuts, and seeds.

The importance of having complete proteins in the diet must be emphasized. Unless all of the essential amino acids are present simultaneously and in adequate amounts, protein synthesis will not be carried out. Not even one of these important substances can be missing, or even supplied later. The indisputable law of protein is all-or-nothing-at-all.

This does not mean that a diet must consist entirely of large amounts of meat, in order for the person to receive adequate protein. Many vegetarians have proven that living without meat can be a highly successful and healthy way of life. For women with menstrual difficulties, it might even be advantageous. **Dr. and Mrs. Seaman suspect that there may be elements in meat which aggravate menstrual cramps because they have found that cramps are rarer in vegetarian societies, and also in American women who cut back on their meat intake.** To cut back on red meat just prior to and during the symptom phase and to rely more on fish, poultry, whole grains, and legumes may prove beneficial.

Independent studies have indicated that, contrary to past opinion, proteins from many vegetable sources are equal or even superior to animal protein in their biological value. The problem is that vegetable proteins are only partially complete and, therefore, must be combined with other specific, complementary sources to form that complete nutrient. The practice of combining proteins is not easy, but neither is it impossible. A few common examples of protein complements are tortillas and beans, macaroni and cheese, pizza, and peanut butter on whole wheat bread. There are many excellent books now available for the person who wishes to eliminate meat from the diet and still be assured of adequate nutrition.

Protein quality is evaluated in yet another way—according to its "biological value." A measure used in determining the extent to which the amino acid pattern of a protein matches that which the body can use is the *net protein utilization* (NPU) value. It takes two factors into account: the amino acid composition of the protein, and its digestibility. In other words, how much of the protein that is eaten is actually used by the body? No one food corresponds 100% with the body's required perfect pattern, but the protein in eggs comes closest and is therefore used as the standard by which all other proteins are measured. Amino acid patterns closest to the egg are found in milk, fish, cheese, whole rice, red meat, and poultry, in that order.(18)

The amount of protein required by individuals is a subject about which there is much controversy. Even the experts disagree. For those who experience menstrual discomfort it is probably best to examine protein intake and make certain that at least the minimum is being consumed. One gram of protein for every two pounds of body weight is considered a standard, but some women may find they need a larger amount to control their symptoms.

Before leaving this subject, it needs to be mentioned that

certain people have difficulty breaking down protein into amino acids. As people get older, the body's ability to manufacture the enzymes necessary for this process slows down. Enzymes react with vitamins to chemically convert all foods into their simpler structures so they can be absorbed by the small intestine. Protein specifically requires hydrochloric acid and other proteolytic enzymes for this purpose. If too much or too little of these digestive enzymes are produced, absorption and digestion is inhibited. Undigested protein produces putrefaction and immediate effects such as excessive belching, "gassy" stomachs, and bad breath. If an enzyme supplement is indicated, one including betaine hydrochloride, pepsin and pancreatic acid is suggested.

Sugar

Dr. Fredericks says that even if reduction in sugar intake is the sole change in diet, that alone will often shorten menstruation and reduce premenstrual tension. Apart from not adding anything nutritionally to the body, an excess of sugar will deplete the body of its much-needed B vitamins. In order to metabolize estrogen the liver takes B vitamins that are in the blood and cells. When there are none left in the liver to handle the estrogen, the hormone builds up. As the estrogen level in the blood rises it puts a stress on the body, forcing various glands and systems to overreact. Dr. Guy Abraham has portrayed what occurs in different systems when women take in sugar:

> A woman is eating badly. Her intake of too many highly refined carbohydrates pushes tryptophan, an amino acid,

into the brain cells. The tryptophan is converted to serotonin, one of the hormonal mischief-makers. It is responsible for nervous tension. The serotonin also stimulates the adrenal glands to produce a salt-retaining hormone called aldosterone. So the woman swells . . . If she also eats a lot of sugar, this in turn triggers insulin release from the pancreas . . . More swelling.(19)

The evils of sugar have been proclaimed in many books and articles. It's primary harmful effect is that it deranges the entire mechanism for controlling carbohydrates. The body is not equipped to handle sweets in such a concentrated form. Because it is forced to overcompensate, many organs and glands experience stress. The pancreas, for example, over-reacts to the sugar in the blood by pouring out too much insulin. The insulin quickly draws the sugar from the blood and stores it in the liver and the muscles as glycogen. This drastic drop in blood sugar causes symptoms such as headache, tension, fatigue, depression, and dizziness. The hypoglycemic state, as it is called, can happen to anyone who eats too much sugar, but the symptoms seem to be exaggerated in women prior to menstruation.

The Senate Select Committee on Nutrition has urged Americans to decrease their consumption of sugar, and to replace it with complex carbohydrates. Even so, food manufacturers are continually adding sugar to everything, including hot dogs, salad dressing, canned vegetables and fruits, natural cereals, and even salt. A reading of the labels reveals the various forms of sugar used: corn syrup, sucrose, dextrose, and fructose.

Salt

In addition to supplementing the diet with B vitamins, regulating protein intake, and eliminating sugar, there are a few other steps that can be helpful in reducing the symptoms of premenstrual tension. In her book *No More Menstrual Cramps*, Penny Budoff, M.D., recommends cutting down on salt and caffeine. Seven to ten days before the onset of menses, one should begin a low-sodium diet. This is one way to relieve the water retention caused by the various hormones. As bloating alone can be responsible for many symptoms, such as tender breasts and swelling of the hands, feet, and abdomen, reducing salt-filled foods will help.

For some women, reducing salt may mean more than eliminating the salt shaker or cutting out tortilla chips. It could involve limiting the salt in cooking, and avoiding foods that are high in sodium such as commercial salad dressings, gravies, canned and dried soups, olives, pickles, ham, hot dogs, buttermilk, cheese, and canned foods of all kinds.

Eating a variety of natural foods that are known to produce a cleansing effect can also be helpful. Some of these foods are parsley, celery, cucumber, watermelon, grapes, pineapple, canteloupe, and asparagus. Herbs have also been found useful as diuretics. Dr. Kurt Donsbach in his *Herbs Book No. 2* suggests juniper berries, buchum parsley root, uva ursi, and horsetail grass for use as diuretics.

Caffeine

Caffeine has been implicated in several problems that specifically affect women. John P. Minton, M.D., recently reported that benign breast cysts disappeared in two-thirds of all women tested when they eliminated caffeine from their diets. (20)

Dr. Budoff experimented with the effect of caffeine on premenstrual breast tenderness. She, along with some of her patients, totally eliminated the drug from their diets. Dr.

Budoff reasoned that if xanthines, the chemicals in caffeine products, contributed to the production of cysts, then without them breast cell activity in general would decrease.(21) Generally, she and her patients felt they did have less tenderness, less irritability, and a better period. Dr. Budoff personally believes that her cramps have been milder since her decision to discontinue coffee.

Caffeine is a brain stimulant that acts directly on the central nervous system and affects the entire body. Initially it gives one a lift: the blood sugar rises, the metabolic rate increases, the heart beats faster, and the lungs work harder. The blood vessels in the brain constrict or narrow as those around the heart dilate or widen. Gastric secretions of hydrochloric acid are quadrupled, and the kidneys discharge more urine. The symptoms caffeine causes—anxiety, insomnia, nervousness, irritability, and shakiness—are all coincidentally similar to those felt by women during the premenstrual week.

The *American Pharmaceutical Association Handbook of Nonprescriptive Drugs* cites 250 mg, or about two cups of percolated coffee, as the maximum dosage a body can comfortably handle; above that, symptoms occur. Of course, there are sources of caffeine other than coffee. It is found also in tea, cocoa, chocolate, cola drinks, and even diet drinks. It is included in drugs such as stimulants (Nodoz), weight control pills (Dexatrim), painkillers (Anacin), cold and allergy remedies (Dristan), and menstural aids (Midol).

Vitamin C (Ascorbic Acid)

Vitamin C and the C-Complex vitamins have been useful in relieving many symptoms associated with the premenstrual syndrome. Vitamin C acts as a healer in practically every condition of ill health. It is so universal in its preventive and therapeutic action that it is often referred to as a medical panacea—if there is such a thing. To list all of its functions and benefits would take a book; therefore, just the ones that relate most directly to the menstrual cycle will be emphasized.

Vitamin C is concentrated in the organs and tissues of high metabolic activity, such as the brain and the endocrine glands (the adrenals, the pituitary, and the sex glands). The adrenals are particularly sensitive to a loss of vitamin C as they contain and use more of it than any other part of the body. The adrenals primarily function to produce hormones needed in times of emergency; however, they also secrete more than twenty steroid hormones which directly maintain the body processes at peak efficiency. If undersupplied the glands hemorrhage and the output of hormones is markedly decreased. Russian scientists have discovered that vitamin C will rejuvenate and stimulate all of the endocrine glands including the adrenals and the sex glands.(22)

Ascorbic acid is crucial to the synthesis and maintenance of collagen, the protein substance which supports the cells, tissues, muscles, and organs. The strength of this intracellular cement affects all areas of the body. If the supply of vitamin C runs low, collagen becomes soft, almost to the point of liquifying. Tissues, cartilage, and bones can no longer support the body and one literally goes to pieces. Many of the typical signs of aging—skin discoloration, wrinkles, brittle bones, and weakened arteries—could indicate a low level of vitamin C.

Impairment of collagen formation can be a precipitating factor in many disorders. Houston neurosurgeon James Greenwood, M.D., found a connection between lack of vitamin C and back pain. Through his studies he found that people who died of scurvy showed a dissolution of the back tissues and vertebrae. The evidence was substantial enough for Dr. Greenwood to experiment on his own hip and back pains. When his relief was immediate and lasting, he began prescribing vitamin C for any back trouble or muscle soreness. Treating large groups of patients with one gram of ascorbic acid per day, he found most of them also gained substantial relief.(23)   Many women complain of back pain along with their monthly cramps. It is possible that their bodies are informing them of a need for additional vitamin C.

Ascorbic acid may relieve fatigue by cleansing the body of pollutants. Vitamin C is a potent detoxifier; it neutralizes the effects of most poisons produced from the environment, such as sulfur dioxide, carbon monoxide, lead and mercury, additives, pesticides, and harmful chemicals found in food. Vitamin C increases the therapeutic effect of different drugs and medicines such as aspirin and insulin; at the same time it reduces their toxic side effects.(24)

Recently, vitamin C has been found to have an anti-anxiety effect which has proven especially advantageous in the biochemical treatment of schizophrenia. Commenting on the beneficial effects of ascorbic acid treatment in his patients, Dr. Carl Pfeiffer reports: "the patients expressed a feeling of well-being. The anxious, tense facial expressions were replaced with a smile and friendliness."(25)   Even among people considered "normal," a lack of vitamin C can cause mental symptoms such as fatigue, listlessness, lassitude, confusion, and depression. These feelings bear a remarkable similarity to those described by women experiencing premenstrual problems.

Many factors increase the need for vitamin C and the C-Complex vitamins: fever, infections, stress, x-rays, smog, and smoking. Also, any biological state which elevates the serum copper level, such as late pregnancy, excessive smoking, and the use of the Pill, will deplete the vitamin, causing a deficiency unless immediately replaced. Estrogen in all forms increases the copper level and the need for vitamin C. When estrogen is at its highest point, the vitamin level is at its lowest. If women were to compensate for this cyclic deficiency, they might experience less discomfort.

It is difficult to establish a universal vitamin C requirement because the needs of individuals can vary so drastically. Even the needs of the same individual can vary from day to day, depending on a variety of factors and circumstances. A review of the literature, however, indicates that a noticeable improvement in menstruation has been observed with the oral intake of between 200 mg and 1,000 mg of ascorbic acid per day. (26)

As one of the most widely consumed supplements, ascorbic acid is available in tablets, syrups, powders, and chewable wafers. A good supplement should contain the complete C-Complex, including the bioflavenoids, hesperidin, and rutin. Because ascorbic acid is quickly excreted it is a good practice to take a timed-release tablet, to maintain a constant high level in the blood stream.

Natural sources of vitamin C include citrus fruits, berries, green vegetables, tomatoes, alfalfa, almonds, and bananas. These foods are best eaten raw and uncooked, for much of the water soluble C is lost in cooking.

Vitamin C supplementation will benefit just about everyone. The famous Nobel prize winner Linus Pauling concluded after a lifetime of study that ingestion of vitamin C alone could result in an increase in life expectancy up to twenty years. That is certainly worth considering.

The C-Complex

The C-Complex, which includes rutin, hesperidin, and the bioflavenoids, are naturally found together with vitamin C and are closely related to it in function. They also possess some unique qualities that are beneficial to women experiencing monthly problems. According to a French clinical research team, bioflavenoids were found to be helpful in relieving pain in some women. (27)   They are also reported to be effective in treating heavy menstrual bleeding and irregular menstrual flow. (28)

It is the primary role of the C-Complex to increase the strength and permeability of the capillary walls. When these minute blood vessels, which connect the arteries to the veins, become too fragile, they rupture and cause blood to flow into the body tissues. The result is swelling, bruising, and sometimes bleeding. For years doctors have used C-Complex preparations to prevent nose bleeds, varicose veins, and miscarriages—in fact, any form of hemorrhaging caused by capillary breakdown.

Anxious and depressed individuals have been relieved through the use of these obscure nutrients. In a study using volunteers, Dr. Carl Pfeiffer measured the brain waves of subjects after giving them 50 mg doses of rutin. He found that the rutin has both a sedative as well as a stimulant effect. In another test, Dr. Pfeiffer discovered bioflavenoids to have the sedative effect of two aspirin tablets or two Miltowns. (29) Women who continually take these drugs risk the side effects, unaware that there is an alternative.

The C-Complex is found in the white rind and segment part of citrus fruits like lemons, oranges, and grapefruit. It is also an element in apricots, plums, cherries, blackberries, green peppers, and rose hips.

Normally one takes the same dosage as the vitamin C supplement. An average level is about 500 mg, but more may be necessary for therapeutic reasons.

Magnesium

Another key element in premenstrual syndrome may be a lack of the mineral magnesium. Dr. G. E. Abraham of UCLA studied the red blood cells of women with premenstrual tension and confirmed that they had significantly lower magnesium levels than women who did not have premenstrual tension.(30)   Magnesium is at its lowest level in women during the menstrual period, and this deficiency may explain some of the symptoms they experience.

Magnesium has a calming effect on neuromuscular irritability. Both nerve and muscle action can be triggered when magnesium is inadequate. The resulting symptoms might include muscle spasms, twitching, irregular heart beat, insomnia, anxiety, confusion, depression, and in rare instances suicide. In a study of suicide statistics, French scientist M. L. Robinet discovered that:

> The comparison of geological maps and statistics establishes in a striking manner the influence of the magnesium content of the soil on the number of suicides . . . It is evident that one doesn't commit suicide because the soil is poor in magnesium. But, those who regularly absorbed a good amount of magnesium salts have a more stable equilibrium, they support adversity with more

calm and do not renounce everything to avoid some sorrow . . . The use of magnesium permits one to support adversity with more serenity.(31)

Magnesium acts as a sedative for many people. Because insomnia can often be traced to a lack of calcium and magnesium, it is logical to assume that the body will respond when these substances are provided. Certainly it is better than sleeping pills. For the sedative effect, some people report dolomite and/or bone meal taken with a little orange juice and yogurt for quick assimilation a most beneficial combination.

Magnesium deficiency is very prevalent in our society. American women normally ingest only half of the mineral needed for optimum health. In contrast, Japanese women have a diet that is high in magnesium and practically free from refined sugar (that is, unless they adopt a Western diet). A study conducted in Japan revealed that PMT (premenstrual tension) symptoms of swelling, irritability, and craving for sweets is very low among Japanese women.(32)   In the United States these are all common complaints. This not only illustrates the necessity of a high magnesium diet, it also reinforces the theory that sugar can contribute to or exacerbate PMS.

Sources rich in dietary magnesium include: kelp, brewer's yeast, sunflower and pumpkin seeds, raw nuts, raw or lightly steamed leafy vegetables, beans, corn, and oatmeal. Many factors reduce the charted amount of magnesium in foods. The refining process, cooking, pregnancy, lactation, estrogen, alcohol, and stress—all increase the need for magnesium.

Magnesium regulates the metabolism of calcium; so if one is taking large amounts of calcium, magnesium should also be increased. Those who consume a lot of eggs and dairy products should note that both are high in calcium but low in magnesium. To maintain a correct balance of the two minerals the ratio should be two parts calcium to one part magnesium. Recommended dosage varies from 350 mg to 1,000 mg. As magnesium neutralizes stomach acidity it is better not to take it directly after meals.

Dolomite contains the perfect balance of calcium to magnesium and is considered a good supplement. Magnesium in an amino acid chelate form is also excellent. The process of chelation facilitates the absorption and utilization of minerals. Within the body, minerals normally attach to amino acids so they are more easily transported through the intestinal wall. Because so many people have difficulty breaking down nutrients, this process is frequently hampered. Chelation simply involves covering a mineral with an amino acid to ensure absorption does take place.

Recently, several PMS clinics have experimented with reversing the ratio of calcium and magnesium, and have found that in some women it is effective. Only trial and error can prove what is best for a particular individual.

6

Nutritional Treatment of Menstrual Cramps and Other Menstrual Discomforts

There are several nutritional remedies that have proven effective in the treatment of monthly cramps. At the top of the list are the B vitamins, especially vitamin B-6. As these have already been discussed in the previous chapters their benefits will not be restated here.

Vitamin E (Tocopherol)

Significantly high on the list is vitamin E. This multifaceted nutrient works in many ways. **As a mild prostaglandin inhibitor, vitamin E can act directly to relieve pain in much the same way aspirin does, but without the unwanted side-effects.** It stimulates the action of the kidneys and the flow of urine, and therefore reduces retention of fluid in the tissues. Vitamin E has also been reported effective in eliminating leg muscle cramps, and in decreasing the breast tenderness and congestion experienced by women before and during menstruation.

Initially, alpha tocopherol, a part of vitamin E, was studied in association with the sexual function. In 1933, Dr.'s Evan and Wilfrid Shute, the world's foremost authorities on the vitamin, experimented with it as a treatment for dysmenorrhea and menorrhagia. In fact, the whole concept of the way in which vitamin E works was originally derived from a study of the pathological conditions that accompany hyperestrogenism, and their correction through restoring the estrogen level to normal.(1)

It has long been established that vitamin E is important both for the adequate production and for the proper metabolism of the sex hormones. After all, it is found in its highest concentration in the sex glands, the adrenals, and the pituitary, all of which are equally vital to the operation of the menstrual cycle. Vitamin E acts to normalize the activities of these glands and thereby reduces imbalances and relieves symptoms. Obviously, the smooth functioning of all these associated glands is essential for optimum physical health.

There is speculation that cramps may be caused by a constriction of the blood supply when the uterine muscles contract. G. E. Desaulniers, M.D., of the Shute Institute in London, Ontario, explains what occurs:

> Where this is the problem, vitamin E, by promoting better vascular supply, reducing spasm as it does in other muscle groups throughout the body, and by reducing the uterus' need for oxygen, will also reduce the pain resulting from this.(2)

Vitamin E is widely recognized for its ability to improve circulation by supplying oxygen to the cells. The integrity of the cell depends on an adequate blood supply. When the oxygen is reduced by pathological changes in the blood vessels, alpha tocopherol will decrease the oxygen need and in many cases allow the cells and tissues to behave normally.(3)

The most prominent characteristic of vitamin E is its ability to act as an antioxidant. It prevents unwanted oxidation processes that result in toxic peroxidation and free-radical formation. As it does this, the nutrient serves as a built-in protection against accelerated aging. Dr. Aloys L. Tappel, a biochemist at the University of California, Davis, reports that:

> Aging is due to the process of oxidation. As we grow older, the oxygenation of our cells is diminished and because of increased oxidation of fats, destructive substances called free-radicals are formed. These free-radicals destroy normal cell metabolism and thus cause aging.(4)

Alpha tocopherol shares this ability to decrease the need for oxygen in the tissues and organs of the body with other antioxidants like vitamin C and the trace mineral selenium. Dr. Linus Pauling has repeatedly commented that a combination of these antioxidants may be the best means for staying young.

Americans today suffer from diseases caused by external stresses such as pollution, chemicals, drugs, and poor food choices, and from internal stresses such as tension, frustration, and unhappy situations. Dr. Hans Selye of the University of Montreal, noted for his famous stress theory, has written that disease is not so much the direct result of these agents as it is the consequence of the body's inability to meet the stress adequately. While everyone is exposed to external stresses of all kinds, not everyone responds by falling ill. It is the individual with the healthy body and the proper mental attitude who is better prepared internally to cope. Vitamin E is one of the basic antistress vitamins. It increases the body's resistance to stress by improving circulation, strengthening the heart, preventing harmful oxidation of fats, and increasing the supply of oxygen to the cells and tissues. **When well-supplied, vitamin E has a subtle, calming effect on a nervous or stressed individual.**

Vitamin E is present in many foods. It is found most abundantly in the oils of grains, nuts, seeds, and in many vegetable oils (corn, soybean, and safflower). It is found in small amounts in vegetables and in eggs. Because it is so widely available, many people feel it does not require supplementation. Unfortunately, this is not the case. Vitamin E does not easily survive processing, storing, freezing, or heating. Frying food in oil, for example, destroys 75% of vitamin E, and essentially none remains in typical "supermarket" refined oil or in refined flour and packaged cereal.(5)   There are also over four thousand additives present in our foods now, many of which contribute to the destruction of the normal activity of vitamin E.

There are four factions of the tocopherols: alpha, beta, delta, and gamma. Alpha is the most active form of the vitamin in its influence on intracellular chemistry but the least active as an antioxidant. For complete protection, one should use a combination of tocopherols as a supplement.

To relieve menstrual cramps the Seamans recommend 30 IU to 200 IU per day of vitamin E.(6)   Some nutritionists increase the dosage to as high as 1200 IU, but the conservative average ranges between 400 IU to 600 IU daily.

A few special facts concerning the vitamin should be

mentioned. Supplementary iron in the form of ferrous sulfate is antagonistic to vitamin E, therefore, it is best either to take the vitamins half a day apart or to take them with organic iron complexes.

A word of caution for anyone with an overactive thyroid, diabetes, high blood pressure, or rheumatic heart disease: before taking vitamin E, consult a physician. Vitamin E can elevate the blood pressure in some individuals because of its diuretic properties. However, if started gradually and with a low dosage, this problem should not occur, in fact, eventually it could even lower blood pressure. (7)

Many people are concerned about the toxic effects of fat soluble vitamins. Even though vitamin E is fat soluble, its chemical action is more like that of a water soluble nutrient in that 60 to 70 percent of it is excreted in the feces. For most people, vitamin E is quite safe.

Calcium

Supplemental calcium has brought relief to many women suffering from dysmenorrhea. It is thought that a part of women's monthly discomfort is probably a result of calcium levels in the blood declining before the onset of menstruation. About ten days prior to menstruation calcium levels drop, and they remain low until the end of the cycle. The decreased blood calcium produces stress in the body, causing the production of cortisone and aldosterone and resulting in retention of salt and water. This alone can be responsible for symptoms like swelling, weight increase, headaches, muscular cramps, insomnia, nervousness, and premenstrual tension. Often calcium supplements can relieve many of these symptoms entirely.

There is a special link between calcium and estrogen, which may provide an explanation for blood calcium levels in the female body declining around menstruation. This connection was discovered when it was found that postmenopausal women, who have a significantly decreased calcium supply, become more susceptible to the calcium-robbing bone condition *osteoporosis*. Apparently, estrogen enables the body to both retain and utilize calcium more efficiently, so when estrogen is not being produced in quantity calcium is not as easily absorbed. We know that in menstruating women estrogen levels fluctuate each month, with the peak at midcycle and the lowest point immediately prior to the period. Reports show that generally water retention is noticed at the time when the level first begins to drop (after the second estrogen peak), and cramps tend to be most debilitating just prior to and during the first few days of the period (when estrogen levels are at their lowest). (8)

Calcium serves as a nerve tranquilizer and helps to overcome tension and irritability. It has been found that there are strong similarities between the symptoms of an anxiety attack and the mental effects of a calcium deficiency. Dr. F. Flach of Cornell Medical Center has discovered that improvement in depression is accompanied by increased retention of calcium in the body. (9)   Psychiatrist Dr. H. Newbold likewise has found that a significant number of his patients improve with calcium supplementation alone. (10)

Not only does calcium reduce anxiety, it also exerts a calming and sedative action that enables people to relax and get to sleep. An inadequate calcium intake or poor calcium absorption is known to cause insomnia. The old folk remedy of a warm glass of milk at bedtime is now receiving medical acceptance because of this fact.

Medically, calcium is used as a painkiller. The various treatments that respond to oral calcium (often used in combination with vitamin D) are labor pains, arthritis, muscular aches, cramps, and menopausal disorders.(11)   While it seems too simple a cure to be true, many women have found that calcium alone has solved their problems with menstrual cramps.

The primary sources of calcium are milk and milk products such as cheese and yogurt. For those who cannot digest milk, other sources include eggs, dried beans, peanuts, almonds, sunflower seeds, and oranges.

The lack of adequate calcium in present-day diets is substantiated by the United States Department of Agriculture. Their survey estimates that over 30 percent of Americans are calcium-deficient. The major problem, other than not consuming enough calcium-rich foods, is that the mineral is poorly absorbed in the body. Actually only 20 percent to 40 percent of the calcium consumed is ever used by the body.

There are several possibilities for impaired utilization. Foods that are high in oxalic acid, like spinach, rhubarb, and chocolate, prevent calcium from being absorbed. Other everyday foods such as cereals, grains, sugar, and excessive amounts of fats also inhibit the digestion process. Too much phosphorus disrupts the ideal balance of the minerals, again causing a similar situation. Maintaining the proper calcium-phosphorus balance (1 part phosphorus to 2½ parts calcium) is not easy these days when phosphates are generously added to food, when soda pop is drunk like water, and when meat is eaten in large quantities. The fact that meat has 22 times as much phosphorus as calcium could partially explain why lacto-vegetarians very seldom complain of menstrual pains and cramps: they are not as likely to have an overabundance of phosphorus.

Adelle Davis has recommended that when cramps occur one should take one or two calcium tablets every hour for quick relief. (12)   If this causes diarrhea, the amount can be lowered. Of course all women have to determine their own best dosage, but three to six tablets a day premenstrually and during menstruation seem to be most beneficial. As a result of biochemical differences some ladies may require up to 2,000 mg per day.

Supplemental calcium comes in several forms. Bonemeal, calcium gluconate (a vegetable source), calcium lactate (a milk sugar derivative), and calcium orotate are all good sources. Chelated calcium is often recommended by nutritionists because the process of chelation enables minerals to be more easily absorbed. Calcium should be combined with other minerals—especially magnesium and phosphorus—to ensure an good mineral balance. Dolomite is a source of natural calcium and magnesium, and bone meal is a combination of calcium and phosphorus. To facilitate absorption vitamins A, D, and C should be taken at the same time.

Vitamin A

Vitamin A has been used in high doses for the treatment of painful menstruation. Its action is said to emanate from the stimulating effect it has on the pituitary gland. If the pituitary is not sufficiently activated to secrete its hormones, the ovaries will not respond by releasing their hormones. An upset in the feedback mechanism often results in imbalance.

With disequilibrium comes menstrual dysfunction, followed by pain and other symptoms.

Like vitamin C and calcium, vitamin A levels in women fluctuate during the menstrual cycle. It has been shown in animal studies that laboratory-induced vitamin A deficiency decreases hormone production and suspends the menstrual cycle. **Research on humans has confirmed the fact that women with menstrual problems suffer from a lack of vitamin A.**

Dr.'s D. M. Lithgow and W. M. Politzer of Johannesberg, South Africa, tested the vitamin A levels in 71 women suffering from menorrhagia and found, on the average, only 67 International Units (IU) of the vitamin per 100 milliliters of blood. By comparison, a group of healthy controls with normal menstrual periods had about 166 IU per 100 milliliters—almost 2½ times the amount measured in the first group. (13)

Utilizing this information, other researchers treated women who had dysfunctional bleeding with 60,000 IU of vitamin A a day for 35 days. Close to 93% of those treated were either cured or helped by the vitamin. (14)   This seems to confirm a strong correlation between vitamin A and the female hormone.

All endocrine glands, and especially those associated with the reproductive cycle, are fed and stimulated by vitamin A. If the vitamin is in short supply the glands perform less effectively. Because all the glands and hormones operate as a feedback system, the reverse is also true. When the glands are not functioning or are overworked, as they might be with a poor diet, the vitamin supply will be minimal at best.

One of the chief functions of vitamin A is to maintain the

health of the glands and epithelial tissues (the skin and the cells lining the passages of the hollow organs of the reproductive, digestive, respiratory, and urinary system). Without a sufficient amount of vitamin A, any one of these organs or systems can be affected, causing problems women often relate to the menstrual period. Skin trouble, such as acne, impetigo and boils, hair and nail problems, sore eyes, night blindness, and weak bones can all indicate a lack of vitamin A.

Vitamin A is a fat-soluble vitamin, and it occurs in two forms. Provitamin A, known also as *carotene,* is found primarily in yellow vegetables such as carrots, pumpkin, and sweet potatoes, and in very green vegetables such as spinach, dandelion and beet greens. These vegetable sources are often overrated however. According to the Food and Nutrition Board "the availability of carotenes in foods as sources of vitamin A for humans is low and extremely variable." The reason for this is that carotene as it is cannot be absorbed. It must be converted into a usable form of vitamin A. Unfortunately, not all people convert the vitamin equally, and some may be seriously impaired as a result. Also, certain diseases and drugs interfere with the conversion process and make utilization even more difficult. Preformed vitamin A, called *retinol,* is found in fish (especially the liver oils), in butter, and in the liver fats of various animals. Because these forms are easier to assimilate, they are preferred to the vegetable sources.

Many factors can contribute to a deficiency in vitamin A: an excessive amount of estrogen, unhealthy glands, stress, inadequate intake of fats in the diet, problems with absorption, and a deficiency in other vitamins, particularly vitamin E. Many studies affirm that vitamin A is a frequently missed nutrient in the American diet. **A nutritional status report** showed 30 percent of the population was below average in vitamin A concentration in the liver; these statistics indicate a long-term deficiency.(15)

The amount of vitamin A necessary for daily needs as well as for therapeutic benefit remains a debatable subject. While the FDA recommends 5,000 IU, nutrition-oriented physicians give 50,000 IU daily for up to six months with excellent results and no signs of toxicity. Dr. E. Cheraskin, who studied the level of vitamin A which produced the healthiest, most symptom-free people, found that for women, 33,000 IU was ideal.(16)

Iron

Gynecologists report that loss of vitality is the most common female complaint. **Especially during their period, women often complain of a lack of energy and initiative. This feeling could be due to a deficiency in the mineral iron.** It is undoubtedly the most widespread nutrient shortage in the female diet today. Each month women lose two to four tablespoons of blood and with it 15 mg to 30 mg of iron. If the reserves are not replaced, deficiency results.

Iron is the foundation for healthy blood. The body uses it to produce over 200 billion red blood cells every day. As a necessary component of hemoglobin, iron is carried with oxygen into the cell tissues. After it binds itself to carbon dioxide it is carried back to the lungs to be exhaled. It is this property of transporting oxygen to the body tissues and removing carbon dioxide that makes iron so vital to the blood. Even a minor deficit can cause a lack of oxygen, resulting in immediate symptoms of fatigue, headaches, and shortness of breath.

For most women, consuming enough iron is a very real problem. Dr. Carlton Fredericks states that it takes 1,000 calories of well-selected foods to supply just 6 mg of iron. Therefore, to get the minimum 18 mg necessary, women would have to consume 3,000 calories of iron-rich foods per day. However, few of the weight-conscious women of today are likely to choose obesity over anemia. Supplementation appears to be the logical recourse.

As with most nutrients, ingestion is only the first part of the nutritional process. Absorption too can pose difficulties, and this is especially true of iron. Iron absorption is extremely complex, and is influenced not only by antagonistic foods in the diet but also by the actual type of iron eaten.

There are two types of iron found in food, *heme iron* and *non-heme iron*. About forty percent of the iron in animal tissues is heme iron and this is the form the body most readily accepts. The remaining iron in animal tissue, the iron in dairy products, and the iron in non-animal sources like vegetables and whole grain products is of the non-heme variety, and is much more difficult to absorb. For example, only one and a half percent of the iron present in spinach is absorbed, whereas twelve to twenty percent of that in veal is utilized.(17)

Iron absorption can also be decreased by other foods in the diet. Phytates found in grains, tannins found in coffee and tea, phosphate additives found in soft drinks, candy, ice cream and baked goods—all make iron difficult to absorb. By forming compounds with the non-heme iron these "inhibitors" render the mineral almost useless to the body.

Iron needs vary. Women using an intrauterine device (IUD) usually have more bleeding and often require a greater amount of iron. In some women the dosage needed may be as much as five times the normal requirement.(18)   For women taking the Pill the standard is reversed, and the need for iron is decreased. It is believed that the reasons for this are that estrogen increases serum iron, and periods are more regular with less blood flow.

The form of iron most easy to assimilate is chelated iron. Other good organic iron supplements are ferrous gluconate, ferrous fumerate, ferrous citrate, or ferrous peptonate. Vitamin C helps to increase the absorption of iron, and the amino acids in protein and the minerals copper, cobalt, and manganese also enhance iron utilization.

Exercise

Exercise is as much a nutritional remedy as are food supplements, and it plays an integral part in the total health of the individual. Physical exercise during menstruation is especially encouraged for women who experience dysmenorrhea. **Any exercise that improves circulation, muscular strength and flexibility in the abdominal region often relieves the discomfort of cramps and lower backache.**(19)   Researchers have found, after studying the menstrual experiences of competitive athletes and gymnasts, that the athletics had a "strikingly favorable effect on the premenstrual syndrome," with a drastic reduction in the incidence of headache and tension.(20)

According to the President's Council on Fitness, 70% to 80% of the women who suffer menstrual problems are guilty of poor living habits—with lack of exercise leading the list. It has been proven that a sedentary life-style contributes to symptoms and diseases of all kinds, while activity promotes good health and a longer life span. Dan Georgakas, a researcher who studied tens of thousands of the world's longest-lived individuals, found that the most common factor in the biographies of the populations studied was the continued strenuous activity throughout their lives. (21)

The exercises most often recommended for women with cramps and for those who wish to prevent the problem from occurring are muscle-toning and breathing exercises. These recommendations are based on a scientifically proven theory that a problem-free menstrual period is closely tied to there being proper amounts of oxygen in the body and a free flow of oxygen-carrying blood to all systems and organs. (22)

Exercise requires healthy deep breathing, which brings more oxygen from the lungs to the heart and distributes it to all parts of the body including the uterus. With a good supply of oxygen and blood, the uterus is relaxed. The increased circulation increases the number and size of the blood vessels that transports blood to the body tissues and thus enriches even more cells and organs. The entire body is nourished.

Both physical and emotional distress are relieved by increasing the flow of air into the body. Women having cramps or other muscle-related difficulties often tense up in anticipation of pain. Their breathing becomes shallow, which starves the body of the oxygen needed for proper muscular health. This puts unnecessary strain on the very muscles needed during menstruation to expel the unused uterine lining. Exercise which produces deep breathing is therefore considered one of the best all-around cures for tension and cramps.

Exercise has been known to alleviate depression and to help people sleep. It gives one more energy, strengthens and

tones muscles, reduces fat, relieves constipation, reduces monthly swelling, produces self-confidence, and can even add years to people's lives.

As with a nutrition plan, any physical fitness program must be personalized. Weight, age, degree of fitness, and individual preference should all be considered before selecting a program. Whatever the choice, it is important that the exercise be regular—at least four days a week—to be effective. And just as it takes time before the results of a change in nutritional habits become evident, so it is with a change in physical activities. The benefits may not be immediate but they are well worth the effort.

Glandular Extracts

In the past few years, glandular extracts have received a great deal of attention. However, even though they are regarded as a new approach for repairing and balancing deficient organs and glands, they have actually been used in the treatment of disease for well over seventy years. The medical literature is filled with numerous case studies supporting the efficacy of these supplements.

To date, the question is not *whether* glandular extracts work but *how* they work. It is believed that glandulars possess small protein-like substances that can relay specific messages directly to target tissues. Writing in a German medical publication in 1972 Dr. A. Kment said that glandular extracts are taken up by the bloodstream and absorbed by their corresponding glands in the body. This means simply that liver extract can replenish the human liver, the adrenal extract can revitalize the adrenal glands, and so forth.

In some circumstances, the use of glandulars may represent a safe alternative to hormone therapy. They are, after all, classified as foods rather than drugs, and generally speaking, one does not have to use glandulars over an extended period of time. To insure correct usage it is prudent to consult a physician or nutritionist.

Conclusions and Recommendations

Menstrual problems should not be accepted as inevitable.
They can be minimized and even cured. There are no miracles
or short cuts but, given the proper care, nourishment, and
time, the body will often heal itself. Good health is achieved
by following certain laws of Nature. When these rules are
ignored, as they are every day by all of us, illness follows. It
may not happen immediately, but eventually the body *will*
react to poor health habits. By primarily eating processed and
refined foods, by breathing polluted air, by remaining inac-
tive, and by leading stressful lives, people violate the natural
process of life.

The body is an excellent indicator of nutritional
deficiencies. While women may not even be aware that they
are nutrient-starved, their body is, and it is sounding the
alarm through aches and pains, anxieties, and depression. Not
to respond to its warning signals is dangerous since this can
lead to serious repercussions. For this reason it is imperative
that women heed the signs that the body provides, analyze
their individual symptoms, and try to improve those areas that
might be responsible for their difficulty. By adopting certain
basic principles it can be done:

* Women must start by eliminating non-foods from their diet—foods that contain mostly sugar and chemicals, foods that have very little nutrient value.

* They should replace these empty calories with wholesome natural foods such as fresh fruits and vegetables, whole-grain products, raw nuts and seeds, fish, eggs, and lean meats.

* Next, it is important to reduce the intake of all unnecessary drugs, sugar, salt, coffee, tea, tobacco and alcohol. They do nothing to feed the body, and drain it of needed nutrients.

* A regular exercise program is also vital for good menstrual health. Vigorous exercise forces deep breathing, stimulates circulation, and improves the absorption of nutrients.

* If at all possible women should find methods of reducing the stress in their lives. Many researchers have noted that when women are overstressed their periods are more difficult and, conversely, when they feel good about themselves, menstruation comes and goes almost unnoticed. It is obviously not possible to live in a problem-free world, and a certain amount of stress is healthy, but one can minimize the deleterious effects of excessive stress by taking specific nutrients, by exercising, and through meditation, biofeedback, and prayer.

* Finally, women need to supplement their diets. This should be determined according to their individual eating habits and lifestyle, the drugs they are taking, the amount of stress in their daily life, and the specific symptoms they have which indicate vitamin deficiencies.

When first improving nutrition, many women do not feel immediate relief. In fact, their symptoms may actually intensify. Hormone production is being stimulated, and the restraining influence of the liver is not yet operating. It takes time for a malnourished liver to respond, just as it takes time for underactive muscles to respond to exercise. The initial feelings are often unwelcome, but the long-range benefits are well worth this temporary discomfort. The transition can take anywhere from three to six months, depending on the person.

The recommendations in this book are based on scientifically proven research. However, therapeutic vitamins do not relieve every female problem or cure every symptom. Some nutrients may work wonders for one person and be totally ineffective for another; it all depends on the particular body chemistry. However, since supplementation frequently works and is safe, it is a reasonable place to begin with a program to promote optimum future health. Not all the vitamins and minerals needed by the body have been mentioned here, and it is prudent before adding individual vitamins to start with a multiple vitamin/mineral supplement to ensure total coverage.

The evidence is overwhelming that nutrition is an effective treatment for premenstrual and menstrual problems. By balancing the body chemistry and controlling the production of hormones nutrition restores equilibrium throughout the body. Symptoms are minimized if not entirely eliminated. There seem to be no risks, only benefits. It certainly is worth a try!

References

Chapter 1

1 Madaras, Linda, Jane Patterson, and Peter Schlick, *Womancare: Gynecological Guide to Your Body*, (New York: Avon Books, 1981), p. 61.

2 The Boston Women's Health Collective, *Our Bodies, Ourselves*, (New York: Simon and Schuster, 1971), p. 32.

3 Lever, Judy with Dr. Michael G. Brush, *Pre-Menstrual Tension*, (New York: McGraw-Hill Company, 1981), p. 40.

4 Gilbert, Charles Richard Alsop, *Better Health for Women*, (Garden City, New York: Doubleday & Co., Inc., 1964), p. 35.

5 Lein, Allen, *The Cycling Female: Her Menstrual Rhythm*, (San Francisco: W.H. Freeman and Co., 1979), p. 43.

6 Maddux, Hilary C., *Menstruation*, (New Canaan, Conn.: Tobey Publishing Co., Inc., 1975), p. 63.

7 Lanson, Lucienne, *From Woman to Woman: A Gynecologist Answers Questions about You and Your Body*, (New York: Alfred A. Knopf, 1975), p. 55.

8 Schaeffer, Otto, "When the Eskimo Comes to Town," *Nutrition Today*, Vol. 6–7:12 (Nov./Dec., 1971).

9 Airola, Paavo, *Every Woman's Book*, (Phoenix: Health Plus Publishers, 1979), p. 522.

Chapter 2

1   Maddux, *Menstruation*, p. 109.

2   Padus, Emrika, *The Woman's Encyclopedia of Health and Natural Healing*, (Emmaus, Pennsylvania: Rodale Press, Inc., 1981), p. 380.

3   Frische, Rose E., et al, "Delayed Menarche and Amenorrhea of College Athletes in Relation to Age of Onset of Training," *Journal of the American Medical Association* 246:1559 (Oct. 2, 1981).

4   Padus, *The Woman's Encyclopedia*, p. 381.

5   "Running Woe," *Time* (Jan. 29, 1982).

6   Lanson, *From Woman to Woman*, p. 101.

7   Davis, Adelle, *Let's Get Well*, (New York: Harcourt, Brace & World, Inc., A Signet Book, 1965), p. 306.

8   Seaman, Barbara and Gideon Seaman, M.D., *Women and the Crisis Sex Hormones*, (New York: Rawson Associates Publishers, Inc., Bantam Books, 1977), p. 171.

9   Airola, *Every Woman's Book*, p. 66.

10   Fredericks, Carlton, *Winning the Fight Against Breast Cancer: The Nutritional Approach*, (New York: Grosset and Dunlap, 1977), p. 48.

11   Ibid., p. 57.

12   Galton, Lawrence, *The Disguised Disease: Anemia*, (New York: Crown Publishers, Inc., 1975), p. 35.

Chapter 3

1   Weideger, Paula, *Menstruation and Menopause: The Physiology and Psychology, the Myth and the Reality*, (New York: Alfred A. Knopf, 1976), p. 47.

2   Budoff, Penny, *No More Menstrual Cramps and Other Good News,* (New York: G.P. Putnam's Sons, 1980), p. 61.

3   Connell, Elizabeth, "Prostaglandins: A New Wonder Drug?" *Redbook Magazine,* (January, 1972).

4   Schrotenboer, Dr. Kathryn and Genell J. Subak-Sharpe, *Freedom From Menstrual Cramps,* (New York: Gulf & Western Corp., Pocket Books, 1981), p. 51.

5   Seaman, *Women and the Crisis,* p. 183.

6   Padus, *The Woman's Encyclopedia,* p. 396.

7   Airola, *Every Woman's Book,* p. 328.

8   Seaman, Barbara, *The Doctor's Case Against the Pill,* (New York: Peter H. Wyden, Inc., 1979), p. 24.

9   Silverman, Harold M. and Gilbert I. Simon, *The Pill Book: The Illustrated Guide to the Most Prescribed Drugs in the United States,* (New York: The Pill Book Co., Inc., 1979), p. 162.

10   Graedon, Joe with Teresa Graedon, *The People's Pharamacy—2,* (New York: Avon Books, 1980), p. 391.

11   Airola, *Every Woman's Book,* p. 539.

12   Nellis, Muriel, "Hooked: A Sobering Report on Women and Drugs," *Family Weekly,* (March 1, 1981).

13   Williams, Roger J., *Nutrition Against Disease,* (New York: Pitman Publishing Corp., Bantam Books, 1971), p. 11.

14   Beiler, Henry, *Food Is Your Best Medicine,* (Random House, Inc., Vintage Books, 1965), p. 11.

Chapter 4

1   Newbold, H. L., *Mega-Nutrients for Your Nerves,* (New York: Berkley Publishing Co., A Berkley Book, 1981), p. 213.

2   Atkins, Robert C. and Shirley Linde, *Dr. Atkins' Super Energy Diet,* (New York: Crown Publishers, Inc., 1977), p. 25.

3   "Dietary Goals for the United States (2nd ed.)," *Select Committee on Nutrition and Human Needs,* United States Senate, Washington, D.C., 1977.

4   Ibid.

5   Reuban, David, *The Save Your Life Diet,* (New York: Random House, 1975), p. 18.

6   "Dietary Goals," *Select Committee on Nutrition.*

7   Turner, James S., *The Chemical Feast: Ralph Nader's Study Group Report on the Food and Drug Administration,* (New York: Grossman Publishers, 1970), p. 99.

8   Williams, *Nutrition Against Disease,* p. 11.

9   Cheraskin E., and W. M. Ringsdorf, Jr., *New Hope for Incurable Diseases,* (New York: Arco Publishing Co., An Arc Book, 1971), p. 182.

Chapter 5

1   Fredericks, Carlton, "The Average Menstrual Cycle Isn't Normal," *Prevention* (December, 1981), p. 29.

2   Fredericks, *Winning the Fight,* p. 23.

3   Seaman, *Women and the Crisis,* p. 131.

4   Passwater, Dr. Richard A., *Cancer and Its Nutritional Therapies,* (New Canaan, Conn.: Keats Publishing Inc., 1978), p. 153.

5   Gayla, Stephen E., "Dietary Management of Estrogen Levels in Women in Relationship to Breast and Uterine Cancer," *Health Express,* Vol. 2, No. 6:19 (August 1981).

6   Zucker, Martin, "Beating the Pre-Menstrual Blues with Vitamin B-6," *Let's Live,* (August, 1980).

7   "Vitamin B-6, Depression, and Oral Contraceptives," *The Lancet,* No. 2:516 (August 31, 1974).

8   Padus, *The Woman's Encyclopedia,* p. 122.

9   Lever, *Pre-Menstrual Tension,* p. 139.

10   Seaman, *Women and the Crisis,* p. 177.

11   Fredericks, Carlton, *Psychonutrition,* (New York: Gross and Dunlap, 1976), p. 84.

12   Zucker, "Beating the Pre-Menstrual Blues," p. 32.

13   Lesser, Michael, *Nutrition and Vitamin Therapy,* (New York: Grove Press, Inc., Bantam Books, 1980), p. 55.

14   Pfeiffer, Carl C., *Mental and Elemental Nutrients: A Physician's Guide to Nutrition and Health Care,* (New Canaan, Conn.: Keats Publishing Inc., 1975), p. 151.

15   Ellis, F. R. and S. Nasser, "A Pilot Study of Vitamin B-12 in the Treatment of Tiredness," *British Journal of Nutrition,* Vol. 30:282 (1973).

16   Davis, *Let's Get Well,* p. 234.

17   Wokes, F. et al, "Human Dietary Deficiency of Vitamin B-12," *American Journal of Clinical Nutrition,* Vol. 3:375 (Sept./ Oct., 1955).

18   Fredericks, Carlton, *New and Complete Nutrition Handbook,* (Canoga Park, Ca.: Major Books, 1976), p. 109.

19   Zucker, "Beating the Pre-Menstrual Blues," p. 31.

20   Check, William, "Benign Breast Lumps May Regress with Change in Diet," *Journal of the American Medical Association,* Vol. 241, No. 12:1221 (March 23, 1979).

21   Budoff, *No More Menstrual Cramps*, p. 73.

22   Airola, *Every Woman's Book*, p. 432.

23   Williams, *Nutrition Against Disease*, p. 187.

24   Lesser, *Nutrition and Vitamin Therapy*, p. 72.

25   Pfeiffer, *Mental and Elemental Nutrients*, p. 134.

26   Pauling, Linus, *Vitamin C, The Common Cold and the Flu*, (New York: Berkley Publishing Corp., A Berkley Book, 1970), p. 99.

27   Airola, *Every Woman's Book*, p. 355.

28   Lesser, *Nutrition and Vitamin Therapy*, p. 85.

29   Pfeiffer, *Mental and Elemental Nutrients*, p. 186.

30   Abraham, Dr. Guy E., "Pre-Menstrual Tension," *Total Health*, (May 1981).

31   Lesser, *Nutrition and Vitamin Therapy*, p. 112.

32   Abraham, "Pre-Menstrual Tension," p. 44.

Chapter 6

1   Shute, Wilfrid E., M.D. with Harold J. Taub, *Vitamin E for Ailing and Healthy Hearts*, (New York: Pyramid House, 1969), p. 191.

2   Padus, *The Woman's Encyclopedia*, p. 123.

3   Shute, *Vitamin E*, p. 87.

4   Airola, *Every Woman's Book*, p. 445.

5   Lesser, *Nutrition and Vitamin Therapy*, p. 98.

6   Seaman, *Women and the Crisis*, p. 198.

7   Mindell, Earl, *Earl Mindell's Vitamin Bible*, (New York: Rawson, Wade Publishers, Inc., 1979), p. 150.

8   Padus, *The Woman's Encyclopedia*, p. 123.

9   Pfeiffer, *Mental and Elemental Nutrients*, p. 272.

10   Newbold, *Mega-Nutrients*, p. 170.

11   Rosenberg, Dr. Harold and A. N. Feldzamen, *The Doctor's Book of Vitamin Therapy*, (New York: G.P. Putnam's Sons, 1974), p. 154.

12   Davis, *Let's Get Well*, p. 247.

13   Padus, *The Woman's Encyclopedia*, p. 383.

14   Ibid.

15   Passwater, *Cancer and Its Nutritional Therapies*, p. 194.

16   Ibid.

17   Weis, Elizabeth, *Female Fatigue*, (New York: Kensington Publishing Corp., Zebra Books, 1976), p. 139.

18   Seaman, *Women and the Crisis*, p. 491.

19   Cooper, Mildred and Kenneth H. Cooper, M.D., *Aerobics for Women*, (Philadelphia and New York: M. Evans & Company, Inc., 1972), p. 30.

20   Weideger, *Menstruation and Menopause*, p. 51.

21   Georgakas, Dan, *The Methuselah Factor: The Secrets of the World's Longest-Lived People*, (New York: Simon and Schuster, 1980), p. 173.

22   Maddux, *Menstruation*, p. 126.

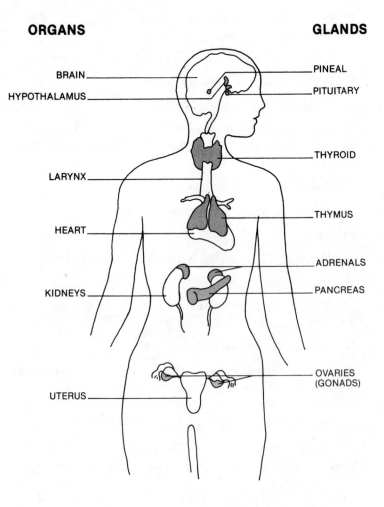

Figure 7   The Location of Glands and Organs
in the Female Body

Glossary

Adrenal glands—Two endocrine glands, located in the upper posterior part of the abdomen near the kidneys, which produce vital hormones. The cortex, or the outer part of the gland, is responsible for the production of aldosterone and cortisone. The medulla, or the central portion, is responsible for the production and secretion of adrenalin.

Aldosterone—A hormone produced by the adrenal cortex which regulates the electrolytes potassium and sodium.

Alpha-tocopherol—The principal form of vitamin E.

Amenorrhea—Failure to menstruate.

Amino acid—A large group of organic compounds, many of which are necessary for the maintenance of life. They represent an end product of protein metabolism.

Anemia—An insufficiency of red blood cells, either of quality or quantity.

Anorexia nervosa—An eating disorder characterized by an intense fear of being obese, a 25 percent loss of body weight, and a disturbed perception of one's body.

Antioxidant—A substance capable of chemically protecting other substances against oxidation.

Ascorbic acid—Vitamin C.

Capillary—The smallest blood vessels in the body.

Carbohydrate—An organic compound containing carbon, hydrogen and oxygen in a particular amount and arrangement. A starch, sugar, cellulose or gum.

Carotene—A chemical made by plants which goes into the formation of vitamin A. It is found in large quantities in carrots. Also called Provitamin A.

Chelation—A process of covering a mineral with an amino acid to enhance its absorption rate.

Coenzyme—A substance essential to the action of enzymes. Some vitamins are classified as coenzymes.

Collagen—Connective tissue around joints, arteries, etc. The main structural protein of the body, making up about one-third of the total protein content.

Corpus luteum—A yellow mass formed in the ovarian follicle which produces the hormone progesterone.

Cortisone—A hormone secreted by the adrenal cortex gland.

Diuretic—A substance that promotes the excretion of urine.

Dopamine—A hormone secreted by the adrenal glands.

Dysmenorrhea—Painful or difficult menstruation.

Endocrine glands—Glands which secrete their hormones directly into the bloodstream, such as the thyroid and the pituitary gland. Also called ductless glands.

Endometriosis—A condition where the cells of the uterine lining become displaced. They can be found embedded and growing on the outer walls of the womb, along the fallopian tubes or anywhere in the lower abdomen. Because the cells have the unique ability to multiply, shed, and grow again under the influence of the female hormones, and since they cannot leave the body, they accumulate as tiny cysts which later grow and eventually form massive scar tissue. It is not considered cancerous.

Endometrium—The mucous membrane lining the uterine cavity.

Enzyme—A substance formed in living cells which speeds up chemical reactions without changing during the process.

Estriol, Estradiol—Other forms of the female sex hormone.

Estrogen—The female sex hormone, manufactured by the ovaries.

Estrogenic stage—The name assigned to that phase of the menstrual cycle beginning at the end of the menstrual period and ending at the time of ovulation.

Fallopian tubes—The uterine tubes located on each side of the uterus. They are the passageway through which the egg is conveyed from the ovary to the uterus.

Fat soluble—Refers generally to substances that cannot be dissolved in water but can be dissolved in fats and oils or in fat solvents. The fat soluble vitamins are vitamins A, D, E, and K.

Fibroids—Benign (noncancerous) growths made up of muscle and supportive tissue found anywhere in the uterus or occasionally outside the uterus attached to another organ.

Free radicals—Highly reactive molecular fragments generally harmful to the body.

Follicle-stimulating hormone (FSH)—In the female, the hormone that initiates the growth of follicles within the ovaries.

Glycogen—Sugar as it is stored in the liver and held ready for release to other parts of the body.

Hemoglobin—A protein in the blood that carries iron and oxygen from the lungs to the tissues.

Hormone—A chemical produced by a gland, secreted into the bloodstream, and affecting the function of distant cells or organs.

Hypothalamus—A part of the brain below the cerebrum (higher brain center) containing groups of nerve cells that control temperature, sleep, water balance and other chemical and visceral activities.

Hypothyroidism—Underactivity of the thyroid gland.

Impetigo—A pustular, inflammatory disease of the skin.

Intrauterine device (IUD)—Plastic material placed in the cavity of the uterus as a means of preventing conception.

Intrinsic factor—A chemical substance in normal stomach juice necessary for the absorption of vitamin B-12 from the intestines.

Lipotropic—Promoting the physiological utilization of fat.

Luteinizing hormone (LH)—In the female, the hormone that causes the corpus luteum to secrete progesterone. It also joins with FSH to cause estrogen secretion.

Menarche—The beginning of menstruation.

Menopause—That time of life when a woman's periods cease.

Menorrhagia—Excessive bleeding during menstruation.

Menorrhea—Excessive menstruation.

Menses—Menstruation.

Menstrual cycle—The rhythmic preparation of the uterus to receive a fertilized egg and the discharge of the uterine lining when this does not occur. It normally occurs at monthly intervals.

Menstruation—The discharge, at more or less regular intervals (once a lunar month), of a bloody fluid from the vagina. This normally continues, except for pregnancy, from puberty to menopause.

Metabolism—The process by which foods and other chemicals are transformed into basic elements which can be utilized by the body for energy and growth.

Miltown—A popular patented tranquilizer drug (meprobamate).

Mittelschmerz—A German word meaning "middle pain." Lower abdominal pain associated with ovulation.

Mineral—Any chemical compound not containing carbon found in nature. In the body they basically have two functions: structural and regulatory. Minerals such as calcium are structural when they form part of the cells or tissues. They are regulatory when they are involved in body functions such as maintenance of the water balance, the acid-base balance, muscle contraction and nerve irritability.

Nucleic acid—A class of compounds found in cell nuclei. DNA and RNA are the most important nucleic acids.

Nutrient—A chemical compound with specific functions in the nourishment of the body. They include proteins, fats, carbohydrates, vitamins and minerals.

Osteoporosis—A disease of aging due to the inability of new bone formation to keep pace with bone reabsorption. It results in a reduction in the density of the skeleton, a loss of bone mass and increased fragility.

Ovaries—The female reproductive glands, one on each side of the uterus.

Ovulation—The process during which a mature egg (ovum) is released from the ovary.

Ovum—A mature egg cell.

Oxidation—The process of combining with oxygen.

Pancreas—A glandular organ extending across the upper abdomen close to the liver. It secretes into the intestinal tract digestive juices containing enzymes that act upon protein, fat and carbohydrates. It also secretes the hormone insulin directly into the blood.

Pituitary gland—An important endocrine gland located at the base of the brain. Its hormones regulate growth and seem to control the secretions of other endocrine glands.

Polyps—A growth of mucous membranes, usually nonmalignant.

Premenstruum—The days immediately prior to menstruation.

Progestational stage—The name assigned to that phase of the menstrual cycle that extends from ovulation to the beginning of the next menstrual period.

Progesterone—A hormone produced by the ovary, concerned primarily with preparing the uterus to accept a fertilized ovum. In general, it increases the degree of secretory activity of the glands of the breasts and also of the cells lining the uterine wall.

Prolactin—A hormone secreted by the anterior pituitary gland.

Prostaglandin—One of a number of fatty acids which stimulate smooth muscle contraction and affect the action of various hormones.

Provitamin A—Any of a number of substances, called carotenes, that occur in nature and can be converted into vitamin A in the body.

Pseudocyesis—False pregnancy.

Pulmonary—Pertaining to the lungs.

Pyridoxine—One part of the vitamin B-6 vitamin.

Recommended Daily Allowance (RDA)—The Food and Nutrition Board of the National Research Council of the National Academy of Sciences makes judgments of daily nutrient intakes thought to be adequate for the maintenance of good nutrition in the U.S. These are value judgments based on the existing knowledge of nutritional science and are continually subject to revision as new knowledge becomes available. Many of the values established are controversial and reflect opinions of only one school of thought.

Serotonin—A chemical found in the blood which causes blood vessels to constrict and contract.

Testosterone—The male sex hormone, manufactured and secreted in the testicles.

Thyroid gland—The endocrine gland, located in front of the neck, which regulates body metabolism. It secretes a hormone thyroxine.

Tocopherol—Vitamin E.

Uterus—The female organ in which the embryo develops; the womb.

Vagina—The female mucous membrane canal leading from the exterior of the body to the uterus; the female organ of copulation.

Vitamin—Organic compounds or chemicals found in various foodstuffs necessary for the maintenance of normal life.

Water soluble—Refers generally to substances that dissolve in water. Water soluble vitamins are vitamins C and B-Complex.

APPENDIX A

Nutrient Supplement Guide for Adult Women

These nutritional supplement guidelines are specifically designed for adult women. The amounts range from a base requirement up to therapeutic doses for menstrual problems. They are conservative estimates, not megadoses, and are established for long-range health benefits as well as for temporary relief from menstrual problems.

There is a base level of nutrients needed by all women, and according to government statistics women are not reaching even the minimum amounts. The reasons could range from the quantity of food they consume to the quality of food they select. It could be that the chemicals they ingest, the air they breathe, or the stress they experience are depleting their nutrient supply. Most likely, it is the combination of all of these. The need for supplementation is obvious, not only for temporary relief from monthly symptoms but also to ensure a healthy future.

VITAMINS

(Base Requirements to Therapeutic Range for Menstrual
Problems)

Vitamin A

Base: 5,000–33,000 IU   Therapeutic: 20,000–50,000 IU

When requirements may be higher:

> Skin problems associated with hormones
> Arthritis
> Low-fat diet
> Malabsorption problems
> Liver disease
> Too many processed foods
> Pregnancy, lactation
> Acne
> Coffee
> Heat (overcooking)
> Estrogen

Special characteristics:

> Too much estrogen prevents vitamin A from per-
> forming normally in body
> Vitamin E is necessary to prevent destruction of
> vitamin A
> Vitamin A cannot be stored if choline is undersup-
> plied
> Synergistic with vitamins B-12, B-2, C, and E

Vitamin B-1 (Thiamin)

Base: 10–200 mg   Therapeutic: 100–500 mg

When requirements may be higher (requirements true of all
B vitamins):

> Taking the Pill
> Alcohol
> Smoking
> Pep pills
> Surgery
> Processed meats
> Too much sugar (high carbohydrate diet)
> Crash diets
> Pregnancy, lactation
> Pre-menstruation and menstruation

Special characteristics:

> Vitamins B-1, B-2, and B-6 work together to pro-
> duce niacin; they should be equally balanced
> Increases the activity of B-12
> Works with pantothenic acid, niacin, and vitamin
> B-2 to release energy from carbohydrates
> Overdose of B-1 can cause B-6 deficiency
> Vitamin C decreases requirement for B-1
> Affects the thyroid gland and production of
> insulin

Vitamin B-2 (Riboflavin)

Base: 10–300 mg   Therapeutic: 100–150 mg

When requirements may be higher:

> See vitamin B-1

Special characteristics:

> Synergistic with other B's
> Works with vitamin A and niacin

Vitamin B-6 (Pyridoxine)

Base: 10–300 mg   Therapeutic: 100–150 mg

When requirements are higher:

> See vitamin B-1
> Inborn deficiencies can make it difficult to absorb,
>   especially in family histories of diabetes and
>   hypoglycemia
> Gastrointestinal diseases
> Irradiation
> Edema
> Acne

Special characteristics:

> Special relationship with magnesium
> Interacts closely with other B's, C, and E
> Needed to absorb vitamin B-12
> Needed to produce hydrochloric acid for digestion
> Take with B-Complex, C, and magnesium

Vitamin B-12 (Cobalamin)

Base: 3–6 mcg   Therapeutic: 20–100 mcg

When requirements are higher:

> See vitamin B-1

Genetic factor may block secretion to stomach
Parasites
Vegetarian diet without eggs or dairy products

Special characteristics:

Synergistic with vitamins A, E, C, B, folic acid,
pantothenic acid
For proper absorption, combine with calcium
Not well absorbed through stomach, timed-release
tablets are a good medium

Folic acid (Folacin)

Base: 200–800 mcg   Therapeutic: 400 mcg–5 mg

When requirements are higher:

See vitamin B-1
Vitamin C increases the excretion of folic acid

Special characteristics:

Vitamin C and folic acid maintain a delicate balance
ance
B-12 and folic acid also maintain a delicate balance
ance
Niacin requires folic acid to be properly utilized
Biotin, pantothenic acid, and folic acid perform
crucial interacting functions on the liver and
other organs

Niacin (Nicotinic acid, Niacinamide, Vitamin B-3)

Base: 20–100 mg   Therapeutic: 40–100 mg

When requirements are higher:

> See vitamin B-1
> Antibiotics
> When calorie intake is high

Special characteristics:

> Works with all B's in food utilization
> Works with vitamins A, D, and C to maintain skin
> Works with vitamins D and E in maintaining digestion and absorption
> Works with A and C in maintaining nerves

Biotin (Vitamin H)

Base: 25–300 mcg   Therapeutic: 300 mcg

When requirements are higher:

> See vitamin B-1
> When raw eggs are eaten

Special characteristics:

> Synergistic with B-2, B-6, niacin, A, and D for normal skin
> Needed to synthesize vitamin C and niacin

Pantothenic acid (Calcium pantothenate, Vitamin B-5)

Base: 10–100 mg   Therapeutic: 100–300 mg

When requirements are higher:

> See vitamin B-1

Special characteristics:

>   Synergistic with biotin, folic acid, C, A, and E

PABA (Para-aminobenzoic acid)

Base: 20–30 mg   Therapeutic: 20–30 mg

When requirements are higher:

>   See vitamin B-1

Special characteristics:

>   Part of the folic acid molecule
>   Helps assimilate pantothenic acid
>   Avoid if signs of estrogen excess, such as premen-
>   strual breast cysts and tenderness, are evident

Choline and Inositol

Base: 100 mg   Therapeutic: 100–1000 mg

When requirements are higher:

>   See vitamin B-1

Special characteristics:

>   Take with other B's
>   Six lecithin capsules contain 244 mg of each
>   If taking lecithin, take a chelated calcium supple-
>   ment to keep the phosphorus and calcium in
>   balance
>   Choline increases body's phosphorus

Vitamin C (Ascorbic acid)

Base: 500 mg–2 g   Therapeutic: 500 mg–5 g

When requirements are higher:

> Infections
> Illness
> Allergies
> Smog and pollution
> Smoking
> Stress
> The Pill
> Aspirin
> Pre-menstruation and menstruation

Special characteristics:

> Needed to absorb iron
> Helps conserve vitamins A and E
> Best taken with bioflavenoids
> Timed-release vitamin C maintains a constant
>   level
> Do not take with Ginseng

C-Complex (Bioflavenoids, Vitamin P)

Base: For every 500 mg of vitamin C, take 100 mg

When requirements are higher:

> Same as Vitamin C

Special characteristics:

> Works synergistically with vitamin C

Vitamin D (Calciferol, Ergosterol, "Sunshine Vitamin")

Base: 400–1000 IU   Therapeutic: 1000–5000 IU

When requirements are higher:

> Smog
> Taking mineral oil

Special characteristics:

> Needed to absorb calcium and phosphorus
> Aids in assimilating vitamin A

Vitamin E (Tocopherol)

Base: 50–600 IU   Therapeutic: 400–1200 IU

When requirements are higher:

> Taking estrogen or post-Pill
> Smog
> Ingestion of too many saturated fats and oils
> Menopause
> Pre-menstruation and menstruation
> Amenorrhea
> Pregnancy, lactation
> Chlorinated water

Special characteristics:

> Interacts with preservatives
> Helps utilize vitamins C, A, B-12, K, folic acid,
>   and pantothenic acid
> Take with selenium to increase potency
> Iron (ferrous sulfate) destroys it

MINERALS

(Base requirements to therapeutic range)

Calcium

Base: 800–1200 mg   Therapeutic: 1000–1200 mg

When requirements are higher:

>Pregnancy, lactation
>Menopause
>Stress
>Lack of exercise
>Working hard in high temperatures
>High protein diet
>Hypoglycemia

Special characteristics:

>Estrogen level affects calcium absorption
>Menopausal women absorb calcium poorly
>Vitamin D needed to absorb
>Vitamin C can aid in absorption
>Ratio with phosphorus 2:1
>High fluoride depletes calcium by increasing excretion
>Oxalic acid in spinach, chocolate, and rhubarb, and phytic acid in whole grains and legumes impairs absorption
>Calcium and iron most deficient in American woman's diet

Iron

Base: 18 mg   Therapeutic: 20–250 mg

When requirements are higher:

> Taking the Pill
> Periods of rapid growth
> Pregnancy
> Blood loss: surgery, donation, hemorrhage, menorrhagia
> Living in high altitudes
> Peptic ulcers
> Colitis and hemorrhoids
> IUD users may need five times normal
> Anemia
> Coffee and tea

Special characteristics:

> Vitamin C enhances absorption
> Copper may stimulate absorption as does manganese and cobalt
> Major deficiency in American woman's diet
> Only about 8% is absorbed

Magnesium

Base: 300–420 mg   Therapeutic: 450 mg

When requirements are higher:

> Prolonged diarrhea, vomiting
> Taking diuretics
> Alcohol
> The Pill

Special characteristics:

> Hormone aldosterone (adrenal gland) regulates magnesium excretion
> Parathyroid regulates absorption
> Phytic acid in whole grains and legumes may impair absorption
> Large amounts of fluoride or zinc deplete magnesium by increasing its excretion

Phosphorus

Base 150–500 mg   Therapeutic: 800–1200 mg

When requirements are higher:

> Pregnancy, lactation
> Excessive consumption of antacids

Special characteristics:

> Vitamin D and calcium facilitates absorption
> Vitamin B needed to be effective
> Too much iron and magnesium interfere with absorption
> Calcium and phosphorus should be equal

Potassium

Base: 2–6 g   Therapeutic: 5 g

When requirements are higher:

> Diarrhea
> Vomiting

Diuretics
Excessive perspiration
Severe malnutrition (fasting)
Surgery
The Pill
Over 40 years old
Osteoporosis
Menstrual distress
Loss of menstruation
Hypoglycemia
Stress
Alcohol
Coffee
Sugar

Special characteristics:

Works with magnesium and sodium
Too little magnesium leads to decreased retention
of potassium
Excessive sodium has same effect

Zinc

Base: 15–30 mg   Therapeutic: 20–150 mg

When requirements are higher:

Infection
Pernicious anemia
Pregnancy, lactation
Overactive thyroid
Excessive sweating
Alcohol
Diabetes
Taking large amounts of B-6

Special characteristics:

>   Vitamin D increases absorption
>   High calcium and copper decrease absorption
>   Works with vitamin A and folic acid
>   Phytic acid in grain and legumes interferes with
>   absorption

Selenium

Base: 50–200 mcg   Therapeutic: Same

When requirements are higher:

>   Exposure to toxic metals (cadmium, silver, lead,
>   mercury)
>   Post Pill
>   Menopause

Special characteristics:

>   Works with vitamin E (take 25 mcg for each 200
>   IU of E)

Iodine

Base: 150 mcg   Therapeutic: Same

When requirements are higher:

>   Pregnancy, lactation
>   Poor soil (deficient in iodine)

Special characteristics:

>   Integral part of thyroid hormone

Manganese

Base: 2.5–9 mg   Therapeutic: Same

When requirements are higher:

> The Pill or any form of estrogen
> Drink a lot of milk
> Eat a lot of meat

Special characteristics:

> Involved in conversion of vitamin B-12 to its active form
> Iron inhibits absorption
> Large amounts of calcium and phosphorus decrease absorption

SOURCES

Barbara and Gideon Seaman, M.D., *Women and the Crisis Sex Hormones*

Emrika Padus, *The Woman's Encyclopedia of Health and Natural Healing*

Earl Mindell, *Earl Mindell's Vitamin Bible*

Dr. Harold Rosenberg and A. M. Feldzamen, *The Doctor's Book of Vitamin Therapy*

Note

IU—international unit

g—gram (1000 milligrams)

mg—milligram (1000 micrograms)

mcg—microgram

A BASIC SUPPLEMENT
FORMULA FOR WOMEN

Vitamins	*Range*	
Fat soluble		
Vitamin A	10,000–20,000	IU
Vitamin E (d'Alpha, Tocopherol)	100–600	IU
Vitamin D	400–1,000	IU
Water soluble		
Vitamin B-1 (thiamin)	25–50	mg
Vitamin B-2 (riboflavin)	25–50	mg
Vitamin B-3 (niacinamide)	25–50	mg
Vitamin B-6 (pyridoxine)	100–300	mg
Vitamin B-12 (cobalamine)	50–100	mcg
Biotin	50–100	mcg
Folic acid	200–800	mcg
Pantothenic acid (calcium pantothenate)	25–100	mg
PABA (para-aminobenzoic acid)	20–30	mg
Choline (bitartrate)	100–300	mg
Inositol	20–30	mg
Vitamin C (ascorbic acid)	500 mg–2	g
Bioflavenoid Complex	500	mg
Rutin	25	mg

Minerals   Range

Calcium (amino acid chelate)	500 mg–1 g
Magnesium (amino acid chelate)	200–500 mg
Phosphorus	150–500 mg
Potassium	50 mg–1 g
Iodine (kelp)	75–150 mcg
Iron (amino acid chelate)	18–30 mg
Zinc (amino acid chelate)	15–30 mg
Selenium	100–200 mcg
Manganese (amino acid chelate)	5–10 mg
Chromium	100 mcg
Copper (amino acid chelate)	500 mcg

Digestive Aids

Amylase activity	15,000–25,000 NF Units
Protease activity	15,000–25,000 NF Units
Lipase activity	800–1,000 NF Units
Betaine Hydrochloride	75–100 mg
Pancreatin (4X)	75–100 mg
Pepsin (1:3)	75–100 mg

Female Glandulars

Ovarian substance	60 mg
Adrenal substance	60 mg
Liver	60 mg
RNA	40 mg
Pancreas	60 mg
Pituitary	10 mg

APPENDIX B

Food Sources for Vitamins and Minerals

Vitamin A Value

3 oz beef liver	45,390 IU
1 cup carrots	16,280
1 cup spinach	16,200
1 sweet potato	9,230
3 apricots	4,490
1 cup broccoli	3,880

Vitamin B-1 Value

1 Tbsp brewers yeast	1.25 mg
3 oz pork roast	.78
½ cup pecans	.51
½ cup peas	.22
3 oz beef liver	.22
1 Tbsp wheat germ	.11

Vitamin B-2 Value

3 oz beef liver	3.56	mg
3 oz beef heart	1.04	
1 cup whole milk	.40	
1 Tbsp brewers yeast	.34	
3 oz veal cutlet	.21	
1 large egg	.15	
½ cup asparagus	.13	
1 oz cheese	.11	

Vitamin B-6 Value

3 oz beef liver	0.840	mg
3 oz white chicken	0.683	
1 banana	0.510	
3 oz ham	0.400	
3 oz beef (round)	0.435	
½ cup spinach	0.280	
3 oz tuna	0.425	

Vitamin B-12 Value

3 oz liver	80.0	mcg
3 oz tuna	2.2	
1 egg	2.0	
3 oz beef (round)	1.8	
1 oz cheddar cheese	1.0	

Folacin

1 orange	45.0	mcg
½ cup spinach	29.0	
1 egg	30.0	
1 banana	27.0	

Biotin

3 oz beef liver	96.0	mcg
3 oz ham	22.5	
1 egg	11.3	
3 oz white chicken	10.0	
1 oz cheddar cheese	3.6	
1 banana	4.4	

Pantothenic Acid

3 oz beef liver	7.700	mg
½ cup broccoli	1.170	
1 egg	1.600	
3 oz dark chicken	1.000	
3 oz light chicken	.800	
½ cup peas	.750	
½ cup lima beans	.470	
whole wheat bread	.430	

Niacin Values

3 oz beef liver	14.0 mg
3 oz tuna	10.1
2.9 oz ground beef	4.4
1 Tbsp brewers yeast	3.0
1 medium potato	2.7
1 Tbsp peanut butter	2.4
½ cup almonds	2.3
½ cup peas	1.4

Vitamin C Values

½ cup acerola juice	1936 mg
1 green pepper	94
½ cantelope	90
1 orange	66
½ cup brussel sprouts	63
½ cup orange juice	60
½ cup broccoli	53
½ cup strawberries	44

Vitamin E Values

3 oz salmon steak	1.15 mg
1 tomato	.60
3 oz beef liver	.54

1 apple	.46
1 banana	.33
3 oz chicken breast	.31
3 oz ground beef	.31
1 egg	.23
½ cup peas	.44

Calcium Values

1 cup milk	291	mg
1 oz cheddar cheese	204	
½ cup ice cream	88	
½ cup broccoli	68	
1 orange	54	
1 egg	28	
½ cup green beans	32	

Phosphorus Values

3 oz calf liver	456	mg
1 cup whole milk	228	
3 oz haddock	210	
3 oz beef	182	
½ cup baked beans and pork	118	
1 slice whole wheat bread	71	
1 egg	80	
½ cup oatmeal	68	
½ cup broccoli	69	

Iron Values

2 oz pork liver	16.3 mg
2 oz beef liver	8.0
1 Tbsp molasses	3.2
3 oz lean beef	3.0
½ cup spinach	2.0
1 chicken breast	1.6
½ cup peas	1.6
1 potato	1.1
1 egg	1.0

SOURCES

Nutritive Value of Foods, *Home and Garden Bulletin,* *No. 72.* Washington, D.C., Dept. of Agriculture, 1978

Eva D. Wilson, Katherine H. Fisher, Pilar A. Garcia, *Principles of Nutrition* (New York: John Wiley & Sons, Inc., 1979).

Index

A Request from the Author

Dear Reader,

I am presently researching another subject of special concern to women—menopause. Some of the specific areas on which I would like to concentrate are:

— Why does menopause affect some women so dramatically and others not at all?

— Do attitudes and stress affect the degree to which symptoms are experienced?

— Can the physical and psychological symptoms be helped with diet, nutrition and exercise?

I would appreciate your help in determining present-day attitudes and feelings on the subject. Would you please take the time to tell me how you feel about menopause? Some questions:

— Are you afraid of menopause?

— Will you be relieved to be free from monthly periods?

— How do you think it will affect your current relationships?

— Did your mother have a difficult time, and did she relate to you any experiences of what it was like for herself and her friends? Did it affect *her* relationships?

Please be as specific as possible. You don't have to include your name unless you want to, but I would appreciate knowing your age.

Finally, as we plan revisions of *this* book from time to time, I would also appreciate hearing from you what you thought of *EXCLUSIVELY FEMALE*, and any suggestions you have for improving it.

Thank you,

Linda Ojeda
Fullerton, CA

AGE
☐ 15–20
☐ 20–30
☐ 30–40
☐ 40–50
☐ 50 +

MAIL TO:
Hunter House Inc., Publishers
PO Box 1302
Claremont, CA 91711, U.S.A.

Use This Handy Order Form
for Your *SPECIAL DISCOUNT*
on Hunter House
Family & Health Books

ONCE A MONTH by Katharina Dalton, M.D.

A clear, myth free book about the premenstrual syndrome, its effects, and complete treatment. The SECOND EDITION has been fully updated with important new information including PMS: LEGAL & DIAGNOSTIC GUIDE-LINES and PMS GROUPS: A DIRECTORY.

2nd Revised Edition   256pp   Soft Cover $6.95

1st Edition   224pp   Soft Cover $4.95

PATTERNS: The Fertility Awareness Book by Barbara Kass-Annese, R.N., N.P., & Hal C. Danzer, M.D.

A clearly illustrated, easy-to-read book that combines accurate information about reproduction with the concepts of Fertility Awareness and Natural Family Planning. Designed and written by experts in the field of reproduction and health care to fill a real educational need.

2nd Revised Edition   112pp   Soft Cover $9.95

1st Edition   112pp   Soft Cover $7.95

EXCLUSIVELY FEMALE: A Nutrition Guide for Better Menstrual Health by Linda Ojeda

This book explores menstrual problems that may result from nutritional deficiencies. With proper nutrition, these symptoms can be minimized if not totally relieved. "Every woman should read and apply the principles of this book." — *Kurt W. Donsbach, Ph.D.*

Revised Edition   128pp   Soft Cover $4.50

DRINKING PROBLEMS = FAMILY PROBLEMS by Marie-Louise Meyer, R.N.

This book provides guidelines for dealing with the problem drinker at home, in the family, at work, and at play. How to help, how to cope, and how — and when — to release: it's all examined here. A clear discussion on the choices that must be made.

1st Edition   256pp   Hard Cover $12.95

See over for ordering & discounts

DISCOUNT POLICY

20% DISCOUNT on orders of **$20.** or more —
A savings of at least **$4.**

25% DISCOUNT on orders of **$50.** or more —
A savings of at least **$12.50.**

30% DISCOUNT on orders of **$250.** or more —
A savings of at least **$75.**

Add postage and handling at $1.50 for one book and $0.50 for every additional book. Please allow 6 to 8 weeks for delivery.

Name_____

Street/Number_____

City/State _____ Zip_____

SEND ME:

ONCE A MONTH (2nd Ed.) . . . . . . ._____ @ $ 6.95 _____

ONCE A MONTH (1st Ed.) . . . . ._____ @ $ 4.95 _____

PATTERNS (2nd Ed.) . . . . ._____ @ $ 9.95 _____

PATTERNS (1st Ed.) . . . . ._____ @ $ 7.95 _____

EXCLUSIVELY FEMALE . . . . ._____ @ $ 4.50 _____

DRINKING PROBLEMS . . . . ._____ @ $12.95 _____

TOTAL _____

DISCOUNT AT _____%   **LESS** $(_____)

TOTAL COST OF BOOKS $_____

Shipping & Handling $_____

California Residents add Sales Tax $_____

TOTAL AMOUNT ENCLOSED $_____

☐ Cash   ☐ Check   ☐ Money Order
☐ Check here to receive our catalog of books

Please complete and mail to:
HUNTER HOUSE INC., PUBLISHERS
PO Box 1302, Claremont, CA 91711, USA

If you don't use this offer — give it to a friend!